A Practical Guide
to Labour Management

DONALD GIBB
MBChB, MRCP, MRCOG
Senior Lecturer and Honorary Consultant
Department of Obstetrics and Gynaecology
Kings College Hospital Medical School
London
formerly Lecturer
Department of Obstetrics and Gynaecology
Kandang Kerbau Hospital
National University of Singapore

WITH A CHAPTER BY
ANNE GREENOUGH
MD, MRCP, DCH
Senior Lecturer and
Consultant in Neonatology
Kings College Hospital
London

FOREWORD BY
A. C. TURNBULL
CBE, MD, FRCOG
Nuffield Professor of Obstetrics and Gynaecology
John Radcliffe Hospital, Oxford

BLACKWELL SCIENTIFIC PUBLICATIONS

OXFORD LONDON EDINBURGH

BOSTON PALO ALTO MELBOURNE

© 1988 by
Blackwell Scientific Publications
Editorial offices:
Osney Mead, Oxford OX2 0EL
  (*Orders*: Tel. 0865-240201)
8 John Street, London WC1N 2ES
23 Ainslie Place, Edinburgh EH3 6AJ
3 Cambridge Center, Suite 208
  Cambridge, Massachusetts 02142,
  USA
667 Lytton Avenue, Palo Alto
  California 94301, USA
107 Barry Street, Carlton
  Victoria 3053, Australia

First published 1988

Photoset by Enset (Photosetting),
Midsomer Norton, Bath, Avon
Printed and bound in
Great Britain at the Alden Press,
Oxford

DISTRIBUTORS
USA
  Year Book Medical Publishers
  200 North LaSalle Street
  Chicago, Illinois 60601
  (*Orders*: Tel. 312-726-9733)

Canada
  The C.V. Mosby Company
  5240 Finch Avenue East
  Scarborough, Ontario
  (*Orders*: Tel. 416-298-1588)

Australia
  Blackwell Scientific Publications
  (Australia) Pty Ltd
  107 Barry Street
  Carlton, Victoria 3053
  (*Orders*: Tel. 03-347-0300)

British Library
Cataloguing in Publication Data

Gibb, D.M.F. (Donald M.F.)
  A practical guide to
  labour management.
  1. Obstetrics
  I. Title
  618.2

ISBN 0-632-01377-X

Contents

Foreword

The last 30 years have seen enormous changes in perinatal care. While many hospitals have produced their own guides for labour management and excellent advice has been provided by the Royal College of Obstetricians and Gynaecologists and the Standing Medical Advisory Committee of the DHSS, there has been no truly practical guide to modern labour ward management. This has now been remedied. In *A Practical Guide to Labour Management*, Donald Gibb has provided exactly the kind of information required by everyone looking after women in labour. It will be particularly helpful for obstetricians in training (especially those aiming to become perinatologists), trainee neonatologists and for medical students with a special interest in obstetrics.

The text presupposes close collaboration between obstetricians and midwives. This is worth stressing because readers in some countries may not appreciate that the provision of high quality intensive perinatal care by a relatively small number of obstetricians in labour wards in the UK and Europe, is made possible because highly trained, experienced midwives care for the majority of women in normal labour and also contribute to the management of those in whom labour is abnormal or prolonged.

A Practical Guide to Labour Management provides clear instruction about modern methods of assessment and practical guidance about effective intervention in abnormal situations. For women progressing normally in labour its philosophy is to provide a flexible approach to management to ensure they achieve the experience of childbirth they desire. The absence of references allows the text to flow smoothly and this is appropriate, for a handbook should be didactic. Adequate guidance is given about further reading. This handbook fills an urgent need for clear and comprehensive guidance and will surely become a classic.

A. C. TURNBULL
Nuffield Department of
Obstetrics and Gynaecology

Preface

This book is intended for all staff involved in daily labour ward management. Medical students and junior medical staff often feel ill prepared when they start working in the delivery suite. The midwife has a wealth of experience from which the prudent junior will benefit, but does not have the more rigorous scientific and theoretical training of the qualified obstetrician. Optimal care is achieved by a perinatal team approach which also includes the neonatologist and the anaesthetist.

Care of the woman in labour is a great responsibility. Reproduction is a basic human need with parents increasingly committed to small families. Anything less than optimal condition of the offspring is an outcome with potentially far-reaching consequences. Demise of the fetus in labour is fortunately an uncommon occurrence today, but morbidity may result in the parents and society being burdened with a child who is mentally or physically handicapped. Natural childbirth is a popular concept, but all childbirth is natural and much of it is uncomplicated. Active birth with participation of the couple is desirable. The role of the medical team is to assist nature where necessary but, more critically, to detect and treat difficulties as they arise. Early detection of impending difficulty may permit preventive measures to be taken: several procedures in obstetrics represent such prophylaxis. Technological advances have provided valuable tools for perinatal care, but it is important that their use should be appropriate.

Obstetric textbooks provide information about obstetric complications and diseases but little on the day to day assessment and procedures in the labour ward. The first part of this pocket size book addresses questions such as the diagnosis of labour, types of labour, the use of oxytocic drugs, the management of pain, fetal well-being and intravenous fluid therapy elaborating a step by step approach. The second part addresses the problems posed by common obstetric emergencies. There is no description of procedures such as breech delivery and twin delivery: this can only be taught in the labour ward. References are not given but further reading relevant to each chapter is recommended at the end.

Acknowledgements

I am indebted to Dr Anne Greenough, Senior Lecturer and Consultant in Neonatology, for contributing the section on neonatal management. Acknowledgement is also due to all midwifery and obstetric staff past and present at Kings College Hospital and the National University of Singapore. The ideas elaborated in this book have been influenced by frequent and rigorous debates. The daily labour ward rounds practised religiously in these hospitals have proved fertile ground for such discussions. Special thanks are due to John Studd, S. Arulkumaran, Sultan Karim, Prof. S.S. Ratnam, Ingemar Ingemarsson, Dora Henschell and others too numerous to mention. Gratitude is also expressed to Sue Gigney, Lesley Elliott and Bobbie Andress for their tolerance and patience at the word processor, to Dr Arulkumaran, Dr Aldoori and Dr Sadovsky for sharing my obsession in finding the right fetal heart tracings and to my wife and children for time spent away from them.

The publisher and Dr Reeders strengthened my resolve near the end which always seemed to be ever more distant: postmaturity has taken on another meaning!

Introduction:
Historical Background

Throughout the world women die every day during childbirth, especially in countries with poorly developed health care systems; they die predominantly of haemorrhage and sepsis. Maternal mortality in England and Wales, which was 5.4 per 10 000 maternities in 1950 has been reduced to 0.8 per 10 000 in 1982; the commonest causes of death here are pulmonary embolism and hypertensive disease. There are many factors involved in reductions in mortality rates. In a historical context improved nutrition, improved socioeconomic conditions, and provision of health services have played a more prominent role than specific interventions by medical personnel.

In the Middle Ages care of the women in labour was undertaken by uneducated female birth attendants. Scientific obstetrics began in 1651 when William Harvey, the father of British midwifery, wrote about labour in his great work *De Generatione Animalium*. During the eighteenth century, Smellie in Britain and Mauriceau in France wrote masterly obstetric texts. William Hunter in his magnificently illustrated work, *The Gravid Uterus*, published in 1774 was the first person to challenge the long held belief that maternal and fetal circulatory systems were continuous and he demonstrated the placental circulation in a wax injected preparation.

The Chamberlen family concealed their secret instrument, the obstetric forceps, for many decades selling a single blade to be used as the vectis in a cruel trick to mislead others. William Giffard records using forceps in about 1726. Recognition of an audible fetal heart *in utero* did not come until 1818. Initial auscultation was by laying a silk handkerchief on the anterior abdominal wall and applying the listening ear directly!

In 1848, James Young Simpson warned of the dangers of prolonged labour. The fungus ergot, which contaminates rye, had been used by midwives since the Middle Ages, but the credit for the introduction of ergot to scientific obstetrics is due to John Stearns, an American physician. In 1807, he wrote that it 'expedites lingering parturition'. However in the nineteenth century a dominant idea was that interference by way of promoting rapid labour was highly suspect. This was embodied in the axiom that 'meddlesome midwifery is bad midwifery'. There was vehement controversy concerning the use of ergot, particularly before the birth of the child; a controversy which was to be repeated 80 years later concerning oxytocin.

Caesarean section was not performed until the late nineteenth century when it was associated with high maternal mortality. The development of the lower segment approach, improved anaesthetic techniques and blood transfusion led to more extensive use of caesarean section after the turn of the century. Contrary to popular belief, caesarean section is not so named because Julius Caesar was born by that method; he was not. His mother was alive when the Romans invaded Britain. The origin of the word is from the Latin verb *caesare*, to seize or cut out. In Roman times if a pregnant woman died, the mother and fetus had to be buried separately according to Roman law.

Sir Henry Dale discovered the oxytocic qualities of pituitary extract in 1904. William Blair-Bell, later to become the first president of the Royal College of Obstetricians and Gynaecologists, introduced it into clinical use in 1909. These developments overshadowed ergometrine, which was isolated and synthesized in 1935, finding its rightful place as an oxytocic after delivery. Posterior pituitary extract had unpredictable effects, which were due to its impurity and route of administration. Rupture of the membranes was not an accepted practice because of the hazards of 'dry labour'. Initially, pituitary extract was administered intranasally and intramuscularly. Theobald in Bradford was the first person to give an intravenous infusion of this substance in 1949. Subsequent developments depended on the elaboration of the structure of oxytocin, its synthesis in 1954 and subsequent commercial production.

More recent research has seen the development of potent oxytocics and uterine inhibitors, the prostaglandins and sympathomimetic group of drugs. Both groups have yet to have their application clearly defined having suffered from overuse in the enthusiasm for early clinical application.

Friedman drew the first labour curves in 1955 derived from a graphico-statistical analysis of labour. Philpott working in Africa in 1972 devised the partogram, drawing management guidance lines on it; the alert line and action line. The action in that case was to transfer the patient with a problem labour from a rural hospital to a centre with facilities for operative delivery. The concept of parto-grams and expected progress lines was introduced into the United Kingdom by Studd. This was an important advance arising in the African continent and subsequently extended to developed countries.

The appropriate use of technology in labour has presented as great a challenge to obstetric staff as the use of pharmacological agents. The last decades have witnessed important developments in electronic technology. The first record of the amplification and re-cording of fetal heart sounds was made in 1952 and since then there have been several generations of fetal monitors. The latest models permit easy reliable recording of fetal heart rate and contractions, externally and internally, at a distance and in close proximity.

Patients themselves have presented an important challenge in their desire to know more about and participate in care whilst in labour. Such a stimulus has forced obstetricians to examine their attitudes and management policies. Every couple should have some kind of birth plan, but this ought to be discussed in the light of an individual hospital's policies. Routine is necessary in a large institu-tion so that staff have a common approach to follow but this may be adapted, bearing in mind a particular patient's attitude or condi-tion. However, routine should not be unquestioning and it is the purpose of this book to outline day to day practice which is safe and practicable. The experienced and knowledgeable obstetrician or mid-wife will know to what extent flexibility is appropriate.

There is currently great concern about increasing litigation in obstetrics. Reading defence societies' case reports, two features are prominent. An event or situation that led to an adverse outcome and an associated serious failure of communication. Often the patient can accept and come to terms with an adverse outcome, but it is the failure of communication that makes them resolve to pursue the issue in the courts.

It is the place of doctors and midwives to recognize problems as they develop and anticipate difficulties in order to prevent them and intervene at the appropriate moment. Drugs and monitoring equip-ment used appropriately in conjunction with basic clinical skills should be powerful allies in the struggle to reduce intrapartum mor-tality and morbidity.

The aim of modern care is the optimum condition of mother and fetus during and after delivery as well as emotional satisfaction for those involved.

Terms and Definitions

Problems of definition inhibit effective communication in perinatal medicine. The International Federation of Gynaecology and Obstetrics (FIGO), the World Health Organisation (WHO), the Royal College of Obstetricians and Gynaecologists (RCOG) and other interested groups have tried to resolve some of these difficulties. The following is an attempt to contribute meaningfully to a resolution of this basic issue of communication. It has become more important especially with computerization and moves towards more comprehensive audit (see Chapter 23). These definitions are not presented as the final word but a necessarily individual and, hopefully, logical view.

Parous having given birth, delivered after a stage of viability, irrespective of the baby being alive or stillborn.

Viability the gestational age after which a fetus is considered as viable should be 24 weeks or 168 days of gestation (RCOG, 1985) (see Chapter 23 for WHO/FIGO mortality definitions).

Gravid being pregnant.

Nulliparous the state of not having given birth at any time. Sometimes confused with primigravid. Nulliparous is a better term for the gravid patient approaching her first delivery.

Multiparous having given birth (by whatever route) previously.

Grand multiparous having given birth on four or more previous occasions.

Primigravid pregnant for the first time irrespective of gestational age or outcome.

Multigravid having been pregnant at least on one occasion before.

Elderly primigravida pregnant for the first time at age 35 years or older. Implies consideration of prenatal diagnosis and other high risk elements such as complicating medical conditions.

Parae, gravidae the plural of para, gravida.

Partogram a pictorial, graphic representation of labour.

Dystocia difficult labour.

Caput (succedaneum) oedema sometimes forming in the fetal scalp tissues during labour. Commoner when excessive pressure occurs between the head and cervix, as in prolonged labour.

Moulding the change in the shape of the fetal skull as it adapts to the birth canal in labour.

Cephalo-pelvic disproportion (CPD) the condition that exists when a well conducted trial of labour fails to bring about vaginal delivery in a patient with a suspect fetopelvic relationship.

Absolute CPD gross discrepancy between fetal and pelvic size making vaginal delivery impossible.

Relative CPD a poor, ill-defined term (see **Malposition**). It implies a 'tight squeeze' but that is not CPD.

Trial of labour a procedure undertaken in a patient with a suspect cephalo-pelvic relationship. Usually a nullipara with a high head. It involves careful assessment and monitoring, oxytocin augmentation as necessary, crossmatching of blood and other preparation for caesarean section. Some would say that every nulliparous labour is a trial of labour.

Trial of scar trial of labour with a scar is a procedure undertaken to see if vaginal delivery will occur in a patient with a uterus scarred, usually by previous caesarean section. The same conditions apply as in trial of labour, however oxytocin augmentation is undertaken with great caution and relevant observations made to detect scar dehiscence.

Pelvimetry measurement of the pelvis; it may be clinical or radiological. It has been done by magnetic resonance imaging (MRI)!

Trial of breech a bad term which should be rejected.

Cervical score five elements of the cervix indicating favourability in early labour or prior to induction of labour (see Chapter 1).

Ripe, favourable cervix a good score; > 6 out of 10.

Unripe, unfavourable cervix a poor score; < 5 out of 10.

Multips os a bad term which should be discarded in the assessment of early labour; simply the os of a multip! Such observations may be appropriate in other circumstances of pelvic examination.

Engagement of fetal head passage of the widest diameters of the head through the inlet of the pelvis.

Fifths palpable of head level of the head in relation to the brim of the pelvis (related to engagement and another view of station).

Free, floating head loose description of a high, unengaged head.

Fixed head loose description of an immobile head which could be engaged or not engaged (better discarded).

Engagement of the breech a clinically meaningless term which should be discarded.

Induction of labour starting labour in a patient who is not in labour with membranes intact.

Stimulation of labour starting labour in a patient who is not in labour with membranes ruptured (premature rupture of the membranes, PROM).

Augmentation of labour attempting to correct slow progress in spontaneous labour, usually using oxytocin.

Acceleration of labour the same meaning as augmentation but a term best discarded because of misunderstanding of speeding up.

Active management of labour a comprehensive care plan proposed by O'Driscoll in 1969, including education for labour, one-to-one care, and liberal augmentation with a consequent decrease in operative delivery and time in labour.

Lie of the fetus the longitudinal axis of the fetus with respect to the longitudinal axis of the uterus.

Presentation that part of the fetus nearest the pelvic inlet and birth canal.

Malpresentation any presentation other than the vertex (e.g. brow, face, breech, shoulder).

Vertex diamond shaped area bounded by anterior, posterior fontanelles and both parietal eminences.

Position relationship of the denominator to maternal pelvis.

Denominator occiput in cephalic presentation, sacrum in breech presentation, mentum in face presentation.

Malposition a position of the denominator not consistent with the stage of labour. Commonly used to mean occipito-posterior (OP) position but also used in transverse arrest at full dilatation.

Attitude position of fetal limbs, body and head with respect to each other. Normal fetal position is universal flexion. Brow presentation is abnormal attitude.

Station level of descent of the presenting part with respect to the maternal pelvis (reference point ischial spines *per vaginam*). Fifths palpable observes the same element from a different perspective.

Asynclitism when the sagittal suture of the fetal skull does not lie midway between the maternal sacral promontory and pubic symphysis; the head is tilted. This causes parietal presentation.

Oligohydramnios an abdomen, usually small for dates, where the fetal parts are very easily felt with the uterus moulded round them; the absence of a sensation of fluid.

Polyhydramnios an abdomen that is large for dates with a tense, cystic sensation making it difficult to feel fetal parts.

Postpartum haemorrhage the most difficult definition of all! Definitions involving volume lost are difficult to apply in practice. There is excessive blood loss after delivery likely to lead or leading to a rising pulse rate, falling blood pressure and poor peripheral perfusion.

Pre-term, premature before 37 completed weeks of gestation (WHO/FIGO).

Post-term, postmature, post-dates after 42 completed weeks of gestation (WHO/FIGO).

Low birth weight less than 2500 g (WHO/FIGO).

Very low birth weight less than 1500 g.

Fetal distress an unsatisfactory term conventionally used to describe a situation implying fetal hypoxia or an abnormal fetal heart rate (FHR). Unsatisfactory because many fetuses with an abnormal FHR are not hypoxic.

Abnormal FHR (cardiotocogram) descriptive term of a CTG which is not normal (see Chapter 11).

Fetal acidosis, borderline fetal pH 7.20–7.25.

Fetal acidosis fetal pH < 7.20.

Asphyxia metabolic derangement during labour, or at birth, associated with hypoxia, hypercarbia and acidosis resulting in Apgar score of 6 or less at 1 minute.

For mortality and audit definitions see Chapter 23.

Part 1
Labour Ward Procedures and Practices

1

Diagnosis and Onset of Labour

Labour is the process of birth. The onset of labour is the onset of painful, progressive uterine contractions, at least one every 10 minutes with or without a show or rupture of the membranes leading to progressive changes in the uterine cervix.

This is the most important diagnosis in obstetrics and should be understood in the context of uterine physiology. The human uterus is active throughout reproductive life, especially during pregnancy. In 1872, Braxton Hicks described contractions during pregnancy and reported their value in its diagnosis. Spontaneous uterine contractions play an important part in the preparation of the uterus and cervix before labour begins; simply palpating the pregnant abdomen may stimulate a contraction and confuse the inexperienced observer. The preparatory time of about 5 weeks before the onset of labour has been called prelabour. Bishop (1964) and Hendricks (1983) have documented the changes taking place in the cervix, showing that the more favourable the cervix, the closer the patient is to the spontaneous onset of labour.

Hormonal changes in late pregnancy play a role in this process as well as uterine contractions with changes in structure. The cervix retains fluid and the nature of collagen fibres changes with loosening of fibres within a softening matrix. Five elements of the cervix are observed: dilatation, effacement, position, station and consistency. Dilatation presents no difficulty (Fig. 1.1) but effacement and its relationship to thickness has been misunderstood. Effacement is essentially the length of the cervical canal from the external os to the internal os or presenting part (Fig. 1.2). The degree to which the presenting part is pressing on the upper end of the cervix and therefore the station of the presenting part are important in the progressive changes. An uneffaced cervix is 3 cm long or more, whilst an effaced cervix has no length. The degree of effacement of the cervix should be described precisely in centimetres of length not in proportions or percentages. Imprecise reporting results in inter-observer variability.

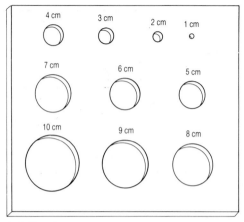

Fig. 1.1. *Cervical dilatation.*

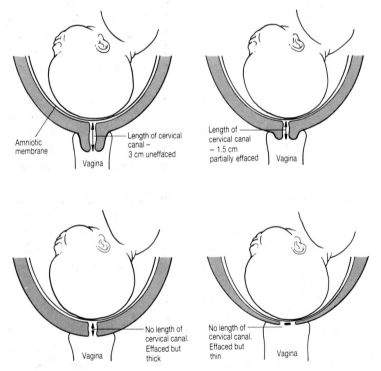

Fig. 1.2. *Cervical effacement.*

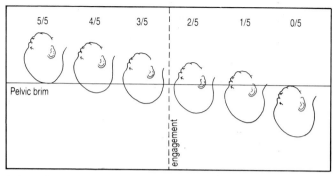

Fig. 1.3. *Fifths palpable.*

After the cervix has effaced it may be either thick and fleshy or thin. Effective dilatation and labour progress is unlikely to occur unless the cervix reaches the condition of being effaced and thin with the presenting part well applied. A cervix is unlikely to be partially effaced and 9 cm dilated. The position of the cervix is the direction in which it faces and the ease with which it may be reached by the examining fingers. Station is effectively the level of the leading edge of the presenting part. It is estimated abdominally and vaginally. Abdominally, the number of fifths palpable of the fetal head are determined (Fig. 1.3) and vaginally the level in centimetres with respect to the ischial spines. Engagement refers to passage of the widest diameters of the fetal head through the pelvic brim and is directly related to the number of fifths palpable. The leading part of a head that is engaged is usually at the level of the ischial spines. The consistency of cervical substance is soft, soft and stretchable, or firm.

These findings will change progressively (ripening of the cervix) with the cervix becoming more favourable as the time of spontaneous labour approaches. Inappropriate favourability early in gestation is a warning sign of premature labour; inappropriate unfavourability warns of delay in the onset of labour and possible postmaturity. This must be judged in the light of the menstrual history, whilst considering the possibility of wrong dates.

Objective scoring of the cervix is useful in some cases when accurate documentation of these changes is desirable, such as in a patient presenting with painful contractions but not in established labour, and in cases of induction of labour. The original Bishop score (Bishop, 1964) is a rather complex scoring system out of 13 and a simple method (Table 1.1) has proved easier to use. The term 'multips os' should be discarded as it is an obstacle to communication without exact meaning.

Table 1.1 Cervical score.

Score points	0	1	2
Dilatation of cervix (cm)	0	1–2	> 3
Length of cervix (cm) (effacement)	3	1–2	0
Consistency	Firm	Soft	Soft and stretchable
Direction	Sacral	Mid	Anterior
Station	Above ischial spines	At ischial spines	Below ischial spines

Score 0–10 if > 6 favourable (ripe); if < 5 unfavourable (unripe). This is a cervical score modified from the original formulated by Bishop (1964), *The Bishop Score*.

Understanding the concept of *prelabour* is crucial to the diagnosis of labour—the most important diagnosis in obstetrics. Prelabour is a 5 week period before the onset of labour when uterine activity increases and the cervix ripens. The painless, infrequent contractions of prelabour develop into a more regular, progressive rhythm. The onset of labour is a process, not an event, and hence there may be considerable difficulty in determining its precise timing.

Labour begins with the onset of painful, frequent, uterine contractions, with or without a show or ruptured membranes, leading to progressive *changes* in the uterine cervix. These will normally be more frequent than once every 10 minutes, but it is the progressive nature that is important. Note that the word changes is used rather than dilatation because the earliest changes may not include that element. Consequently, in difficult cases the same observer must make these observations to reach a conclusion. Pain alone is not enough to diagnose labour and it is common for young, anxious patients to present several times with pain before labour starts. This has been called false labour but is better termed *painful prelabour*. These patients have a low pain threshold which a full history may suggest and is often associated with difficult social and domestic circumstances. There is limited evidence of an association between this condition and a poor fetal outcome if no other risk factors are present. Therefore, mild analgesia and reassurance is the appropriate management avoiding artificial rupture of the membranes, although some have suggested more active management. The possibility of abdominal pain arising from an organ other than the uterus should not be forgotten.

A show, the loss of a blood-stained mucus plug, is not enough to diagnose labour, especially after preceding vaginal examination. Critical analysis of the history is important, as the loss of the blood-stained mucus plug is something of little consequence, whilst a small antepartum haemorrhage is much more important. A report of a repeated show suggests haemorrhage. Rupture of the membranes has a similar significance to a show under these circumstances. It can occur at any stage of pregnancy in the presence or absence of labour. In the latter circumstances, it is called *premature rupture of the membranes*. A show or ruptured membranes in the presence of painful, progressive contractions suggests that labour is in progress. However, progressive cervical changes are critical to the diagnosis.

Diagnosing labour is very important because once that situation exists there is greater risk to the fetus. Artificial rupture of membranes may be performed, continuous monitoring will be considered, analgesia may be appropriate and other management decisions may be made.

Objectively, labour can only be diagnosed after the woman is admitted to hospital. The length of the observed first stage of labour is intimately related to cervical dilatation on admission. Scientific studies of labour refer to the 'observed first stage'. Documentation of the first stage of labour in the clinical notes should not use a retrospective historical observation of when pain started at home as the reference point, but the woman's admission to hospital. The concept of average length of the first stage of labour as described in traditional textbooks is meaningless without a statement about cervical dilatation on admission. A woman who has a cervix 9 cm dilated on admission should deliver quite quickly.

2

Record Keeping

In 1965, Philpott proposed the use of a partogram or graphic representation of progress in labour, the value of which was particularly apparent in the rural African context where he worked. The primary aim was to plot labour progress, detect abnormal progress and transfer the patient when necessary to a hospital where facilities for operative delivery existed. The purpose of identifying abnormal progress will be considered further in the later chapter on the management of spontaneous labour.

Partogram means picture of labour and a comprehensive one will include all the recordings relevant to management. They were introduced by Studd to the United Kingdom where their use has become widespread although this is not the case in America.

The value of a partogram may be summarized as follows:

1 Clarity of recording
2 Clear time sequence
3 Diagnosis of abnormal labour progress
4 Ease of handover when changing staff
5 Educational
6 Research

A completed partogram is shown in Fig. 2.3, with full details of fetal and maternal condition. The basic characteristics of the patient appear at the top: her name, number, parity, civil status and most important of all, special instructions. The type of information appearing in this box would be, for example, trial of caesarean section scar, breech, twins, short stature, etc. The symphysis fundal height and fetal weight estimated clinically are recorded. Below this is the fetal heart rate, and in the relevant space, maternal blood pressure and maternal pulse rate. Below this is a column for maternal temperature, and the next panel is the most important of all with cervical dilatation from 0 to 10 cm and abdominal descent of the fetal head in fifths palpable. A nomogram is traced here using the Studd stencil (Fig. 2.1).

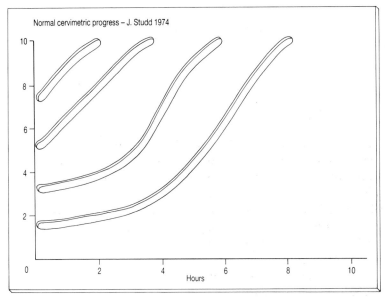

Fig. 2.1. *Studd stencil.*

The time axis is in the middle of the page with particular note being made of vaginal examinations and the times at which they were done. Relevant findings on vaginal examination all have a space below. Oxytocin dosage should be recorded in the space above the contractions panel which is coded according to Fig. 2.2. There is not enough space for intrauterine pressure measurements, but the presence of an intrauterine catheter is marked below the contraction panel. The rest of the printed side is self-explanatory. The back of the sheet is usually blank and should be used to write more detailed notes. The use of a stamp for vaginal examination becomes redundant with this document and more copious recording on continuation pages is unnecessary. Subsequently all relevant information concerning labour may be recovered from this single sheet.

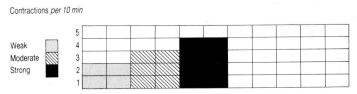

Fig. 2.2. *Contraction code panel.*

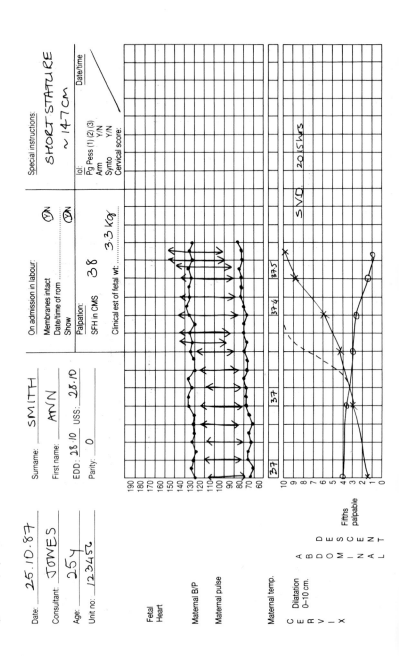

Date: 25.10.87

Surname: SMITH

Consultant: JONES

First name: ANN

Age: 25y

EDD: 28.10   USS: 28.10

Unit no: 123456

Parity: 0

On admission in labour:

Membranes intact — Y/N

Date/time of rom ....

Show — Y/N

Palpation:

SFH in CMS — 38

Clinical est of fetal wt: .... 3.3 Kg

Special instructions:

SHORT STATURE ~ 147 CM

IoI:
Pg Pess (1) (2) (3)
Arm — Y/N
Synto — Y/N
Cervical score:

Date/time

SVD. 2015 hrs

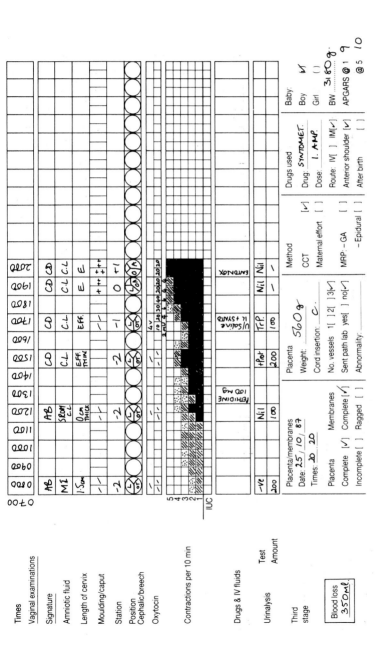

Fig. 2.3. *Partogram.*

Whether or not the Studd stencil is used, and independent of attitudes to abnormal labour, the graphic representation of labour observations on a partogram represents a considerable improvement on numerous pages of long-hand records.

3

Environment and Posture

Women feel more at ease in an environment that is homely and not like an operating theatre or a laboratory. Ideally, the woman should remain in the same room during labour. Transfer from a so-called first stage room to a second stage room is unreasonable at this uncomfortable stage. There are, therefore, the apparently conflicting aims of having a homely comfortable room and one in which obstetric procedures, delivery and resuscitation of the neonate may be undertaken in safety. A better concept of use in planning new delivery units is a low-risk room and a high-risk room or, ideally, a room easily converted for both functions. Attention to interior decoration, hanging pictures and the provision of a radio or cassette recorder make some difference. Modern beds are available which are readily converted from an apparently ordinary bed to a delivery couch complete with lithotomy poles and removable headboard. Good lighting, oxygen supply and suction apparatus are indispensible.

A more important element of the environment is the human one. Women should be encouraged to have one partner of their choice present during labour; children, however, should be discouraged. In an ideal world, the woman admitted in labour would meet a member of staff she already knows. This is not usually possible. Midwives and doctors should, however, introduce themselves, and labour ward staff should consider the possibility of having an introduction board for staff photographs at the admission desk. Personal contact is important to allay anxiety, provide encouragement and reduce analgesia requirements. The most likely and appropriate providers of immediate care are the trained midwife, student midwife or medical student.

Which posture should the woman adopt during labour? This depends on the attitude of the woman, level of risk and any consequent effect on ability to monitor the fetal heart appropriately. Mobility should be encouraged in late prelabour and early labour. There are conflicting reports on its benefit on the progress of labour.

13

However, it discourages over-zealous attention to prelabour contractions and consequent injudicious rupture of the membranes. It may also improve the quality of uterine contractions. If the woman is low-risk, ambulation does no harm and women often prefer it. Individual satisfaction is an important aspect, even though evidence linking it to good labour progress is inconclusive. The questions of posture and fetal monitoring in labour are inevitably linked, and monitoring will be considered in a later chapter. The latest generation of fetal monitors permit effective external monitoring, sometimes of better quality than internal monitoring. However, the woman with a fetal scalp electrode is freer to adopt a squatting, kneeling or other less orthodox delivery posture. Unfortunately, the woman wishing to adopt such postures often does not desire internal monitoring. A variety of birth stools,chairs and frames are favoured by some women. There is limited evidence that they contribute to easier delivery, and they are associated with more perineal tears and slightly increased blood loss at delivery, however, this may not be of material importance. If the use of her chosen posture makes the woman more comfortable and relaxed this in itself is desirable. The partner, or alternative support person, should be encouraged to be present at the delivery as long as problems are not anticipated. This applies to normal deliveries, assisted deliveries and caesarean sections performed under epidural anaesthesia.

The birth should be seen as an intimate event for the parents, and numbers of observing staff limited to a minimum. This may prove difficult in a teaching hospital, but such consideration will be appreciated by the parents. Special arrangements may be necessary for patients with unusual birth plans.

BIRTH PLANS

It is normal and entirely appropriate that couples have birth plans. Couples who do are generally intelligent and sensible, simply wishing to be informed and consulted about progress and events. They may make unusual requests, but are ultimately concerned for the safety of the fetus and the plan usually includes a statement of their willingness to co-operate with any medical intervention deemed necessary in difficult situations. The commonest point of contention is electronic monitoring, which is intimately related to posture. Risk assessment is useful; fetal size, amniotic fluid volume and colour, history of fetal movement pattern and admission cardiotocograph are all critical. Low-risk permits intermittent monitoring with confidence. There is a spectrum of intermittent monitoring: auscultated, audible with machine, length of strip of tracing, etc. Some printed out strip of tracing is desirable to assess variability which cannot be heard (see Chapter 11).

Each hospital should formulate a *Guide to Labour* to inform the woman about events in the labour ward which will help to allay anxiety and limit the number of individual birth plans the women need to prepare. Women's plans often show lack of knowledge about procedures, such as the enema, which is falling into disuse. The *Guide to Labour* (in the form of a letter) used at Kings College Hospital is shown below.

GUIDE TO LABOUR

You will have looked forward to the birth of your baby for a long time, and we hope that your labour and delivery will be both satisfying and safe. We are there to support you and to give you any special help you may need.

We prefer your labour to start naturally; on some occasions induction of labour may be necessary to safeguard your health or that of your baby.

One person, a member of the labour ward team, will look after you. A student midwife or medical student working under the supervision of a midwife is the most likely supporter to stay with you and to help you through your labour.

You may like to think about and discuss some of the following with your antenatal midwife:

- Your husband or a friend may remain with you throughout your stay in the labour ward.
- Most women do not need an enema or shave.
- We may like to listen to your baby through a belt monitor for about 20 minutes when you first arrive, to ensure he/she is well. This may be repeated every 2 hours during your labour. We will listen to the baby's heart beat with the trumpet in between. If there are any special problems we advise monitoring the baby's heart beat all the time.
- We believe it is a good thing to walk around in early labour.

You can then take up the positions that you find most comfortable.

● We may need to break the membranes to look at the amniotic fluid to assess your baby's condition. At this time we may begin to record your baby's heart beat using an internal lead. This may be more comfortable for you, and is easier for us. It need not stop you from moving about your room.

● Midwives are trained to help mothers cope with painful contractions, using methods ranging from back massage to epidurals. Please talk to your antenatal midwife about pain relief and she will record your wishes in your notes.

● Most babies are delivered naturally by their mother's effort; forceps deliveries or caesarean sections may sometimes be necessary to safeguard the health of mother or baby.

● We advise a small cut (episiotomy) if the skin around the birth opening is going to tear badly, but we shall not do so unless it is necessary.

● An injection (Syntometrine—to reduce the blood loss while the afterbirth is being delivered) is given to you as your baby is being born, unless you express a strong wish for this not to be done.

● Nearly all babies like to suckle after delivery; if you would like to put your baby to the breast we will help you.

Please do not hesitate to ask your midwife or doctor about anything to do with your pregnancy, labour or postnatal period.

Individual birth plans should be read, discussed and signed by senior staff in the antenatal clinic. They should also be read and discussed by labour ward staff on admission. Ignoring a couple's birth plan does not generate confidence.

Modern maternity care aims for emotional satisfaction for the couple as well as safety for mother and fetus. The former aim is often denied to mothers in developing countries because of difficulty in fulfilling the primary aim of safety on account of limited resources.

4

Examination of the Woman in Labour

Labour is an intimate and often stressful time for the woman and her partner. Women should be encouraged to have at least one adult of their choice accompanying them in labour. There is some evidence that adrenaline released by the anxious woman inhibits uterine contractions, but there have been no controlled studies implicating this as a major factor contributing to poor progress in labour. Nonetheless, every opportunity should be taken to reassure and encourage the labouring mother. Medical and midwifery staff should introduce themselves personally when they become involved and, before examination, they should explain what they are about to do. Women in the later stages of labour do not appreciate many individuals round the bed, so numbers of staff should be limited. This does not mean that a detailed review of the case should not be undertaken on a regular ward round, but it should be done outside the room.

A detailed general examination is not appropriate and will probably have been performed at an earlier stage. Taking the woman's hand and radial pulse establishes physical contact and permits measurement of the heart rate, a good indicator of overall maternal condition. The woman is then asked if she has had, is having, or is about to have, a painful contraction. If she is having one, the examining hand should be placed gently between the umbilicus and fundus to time it. Examination starts with inspection, and the following should be sought:

1 Contour of the distended abdomen
2 A contraction may be observed as a coming forward of the distended abdomen
3 Pigmentation, *linea nigra*
4 Stretch marks, *striae gravidarum*
5 Surgical scars, especially suprapubic and laparoscopic
6 Fetal movements

Having established confidence with the woman, palpation should then be undertaken to document the following:

1 Symphysis fundal height
2 Lie of the fetus
3 Presentation
4 Station (fifths palpable)
5 Estimate of amniotic fluid volume
6 Estimate of fetal weight

   Abdominal examination is completed with auscultation of the fetal heart. Several elements of palpation require further explanation:

Symphysis fundal height (Figs 4.1 & 4.2). This measurement (in centimetres) has become established as a good clinical method to detect intrauterine growth retardation. It should not be more than 2 cm less than the number of weeks' gestation until 36 weeks and not more than 3 cm less thereafter.

Estimated fetal weight. This is not very accurate but should be done to foster an awareness amongst attending staff of the dangers of labour when the baby is excessively large, especially in the short patient or the small and potentially compromised (intrauterine growth retardation—IUGR). Greater accuracy in this technique comes with experience. An entirely appropriate focus on the problems

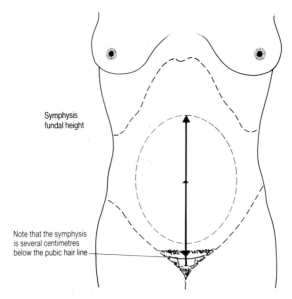

Symphysis
fundal height

Note that the symphysis
is several centimetres
below the pubic hair line

Fig. 4.1. *Symphysis fundal height.*

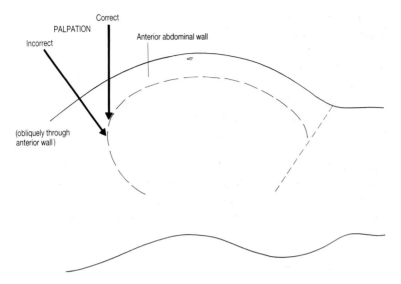

Fig. 4.2. *Symphysis fundal height.*

of the small baby has deflected awareness from, and attention to, the large baby. Large babies still appear too often in the neonatal intensive care unit as a result of intrapartum difficulties.

Estimated amniotic fluid volume. When this is thought to be reduced, especially with a small baby or reduced symphysis fundal height, it is an important associated sign of IUGR and potential asphyxia. If no fluid is obtained when the membranes are ruptured artificially, the implication is the same.

Station. The original concept of station was one of engagement of the fetal head and level of the leading edge of the presenting part with reference to the ischial spines *per vaginam.* Crichton, working in Africa, proposed the use of fifths palpable of the fetal head *per abdomen* (see Fig. 1.3). This has the advantage that it measures how much of the head has still to enter the pelvis. Caput and moulding may make a difference to the level of the head felt vaginally, leading to a mistaken impression of descent having taken place. Engagement occurs when the widest part of the head enters the pelvic brim: i.e. the head is 2/5 palpable. Usually this means that an unmoulded head is at the level of the ischial spines as determined vaginally.

Sequential detailed abdominal examination is inappropriate

throughout labour. However, staff taking over care should satisfy themselves, especially by confirming estimated fetal size.

Engagement of the breech cannot be described in the same way and is a term best discarded. The breech may be described as above the brim of the pelvis, or settling in the brim. It may be difficult to determine the position of the legs in breech presentation.

VAGINAL EXAMINATION

This should always be preceded by abdominal examination and should be done at intervals in labour, depending on the clinical situation. Four-hourly examination in labour is appropriate under normal circumstances, but it may be done more frequently (see below). Provided that labour does not go on too long, too few vaginal examinations may result in more harm than too many. Some centres practise rectal examination but the information gained is less reliable, patients find it less acceptable, and a reduction in the risk of infection has never been proven. Vaginal examination should be performed as a clean procedure; the vagina can never be sterile. Elaborate gowning, draping and the use of masks is unnecessary.

The woman is reassured and, if appropriate, should pass urine before examination. During examination a systematic account of the following should be given:

1 Cervical dilatation
2 Cervical effacement and thickness
3 Application of the presenting part
4 State of the membranes
5 Colour and volume of amniotic fluid draining
6 Position of the presenting part
7 Caput (thickening of skin and subcutaneous tissues)
8 Moulding:
   grade 0: none
   grade 1: sutures touching but easily separable
   grade 2: sutures overlapping but separable
   grade 3: sutures fixed and overlapping
9 Station of the presenting part with respect to the ischial spines.

If there is arrest of cervical dilatation, short stature, large baby or previous caesarean section, clinical pelvimetry should be performed. To the inexperienced, this is not accurate or easy but an attempt should be made to judge:

1 Diagonal conjugate; ability to reach sacral promontory
2 Sacral curve
3 Prominence of tip of sacrum and coccyx
4 Prominence of ischial spines
5 Subpubic angle
6 Soft-tissue resistance

The shape of the pelvic inlet is extremely difficult to judge clinically. Persistent direct occipito-posterior (OP) position and face-to-pubis delivery suggests an anthropoid pelvis. Persistent oblique OP position and second stage difficulties suggests an android pelvis.

Position of the occiput (or sacrum, if breech) can only be accurately determined on vaginal examination. This is shown in Fig. 4.3. Most fetal heads only undergo 90° of rotation during labour, passing transversely through the pelvic inlet, and delivering with the occiput anteriorly passing under the subpubic arch.

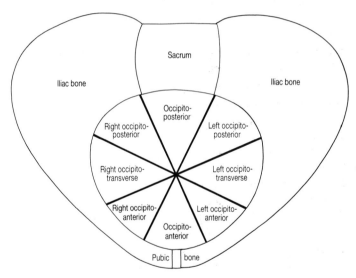

Fig. 4.3. *Position of denominator.*

After vaginal examination is complete, the fetal heart should be auscultated. The findings should be explained to the woman, analgesia discussed, reassurance given, and she should be advised to lie on her side, sit up or adopt the posture most suitable to her.

The final statement in the labour record should be an indication of when the next examination should be performed and by whom. Midwives will usually perform four-hourly examinations in low-risk labour but a doctor and midwife together should examine problem cases more frequently.

5

Assessment of Labour Progress

Labour may start in three ways:
1 Spontaneously
2 By induction (see Chapter 9)
3 By stimulation after premature membrane rupture (see Chapter 9).
The assessment of labour progress in spontaneous labour is dependent on the diagnosis having been made previously. In most cases this will have been done on admission to the labour ward when a diagnosis of labour has been considered likely. In a few cases this will have been a mistaken diagnosis and, if the membranes have not been ruptured, this does not matter. Such a patient should have the observations discontinued and await spontaneous labour as long as no risk factors are present.

A partogram should be commenced when patients are admitted to the labour ward, but a line of expected progress should not be drawn until labour is diagnosed. The mean rate of cervical dilatation is about 1 cm per hour in the active phase. A line representing this is easily drawn across the squares on a partogram from admission dilatation. Alternatively, a stencil of nomograms (as devised by Studd) may be used to draw an actual curve (see Fig. 2.2). This assumes the partogram chart used has the same scale as the stencil. These lines are only guides to diagnose abnormal progress of spontaneous labour. They have no such relevance in induced labour.

ABNORMAL LABOUR PROGRESS

Failure to progress in spontaneous labour may be due to faults in the powers, passages or passenger. However, after early imprudent membrane rupture, the cervical or uterine readiness may be at fault. In induced labour, slower progress is anticipated, especially if the cervix is unfavourable at the time of induction. It should be remembered that projected labour curves have been constructed for, and are only relevant to spontaneous labour. Progress is deemed abnormal

23

in spontaneous labour if it does not fall within certain limits. One method of determining these limits is to permit deviation of progress up to 2 hours to the right of the nomogram before it is considered abnormal. Using this criterion, about 20% of spontaneous nulliparous labours are abnormal. If *any* deviation from the mean is considered abnormal, then this figure will be about 50%.

Three types of abnormal labour progress exist:

1 *Prolonged latent phase* (Fig. 5.1): This is an uncommon pattern, usually observed in induced labour, or labour stimulated after premature membrane rupture. Observed labour begins when the patient is admitted to the labour ward. In spontaneous labour, the cervix is

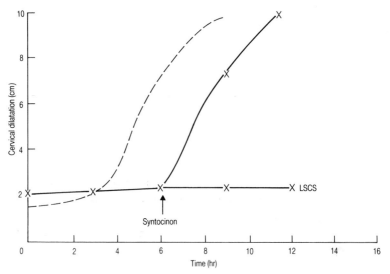

Fig. 5.1. *Prolonged latent phase.*

usually already 3 cm dilated; the latent phase has taken place outside hospital. If a diagnosis of labour is made and yet the cervix remains less than 3 cm dilated for 6 hours then this is a prolonged latent phase. Effacement, direction and thickness of the cervix should be noted; a cervical score may be useful. Intervention with artificial membrane rupture and oxytocin augmentation seems to be related to a difficult labour and the alternative of effective pain relief, reassurance and conservatism is preferable.

2 *Primary dysfunctional labour* (Fig. 5.2): This is defined as being present when no period of normal labour progress has been observed.

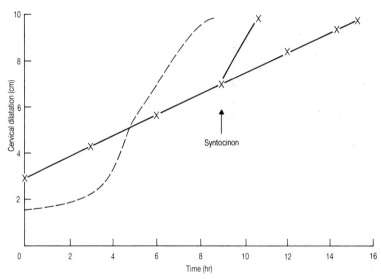

Fig. 5.2. *Primary dysfunctional labour.*

3 *Secondary arrest of labour* (Fig. 5.3): This is defined when a period of normal labour progress has been present with subsequent slowing or arrest of dilatation.

Whilst, physiologically, faults may lie with the powers, passages or passenger the possible clinical problems are:
1 Inefficient uterine action
2 Cephalo-pelvic disproportion
3 Occipito-posterior position
4 Malpresentation
5 Rarely, cervical causes

Careful assessment should be undertaken to delineate which of these are contributory, so that treatment is appropriate. This is particularly important in multiparous patients. Treating abnormal labour progress with oxytocin without considering the underlying cause is like treating anaemia with blood transfusion without investigation. Failure to progress in labour should not appear as a primary indication in the caesarean section register. The nature of the contractions, the

Chapter 5

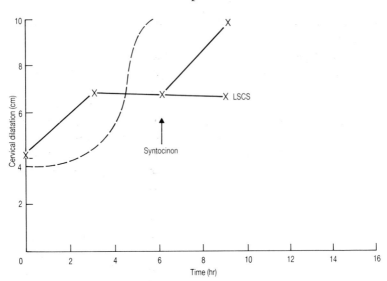

Fig. 5.3. *Secondary arrest of labour.*

feto-pelvic relationship, the position of the occiput, and the condition of the cervix should all be documented.

Poor contractions may be painful, whilst good contractions may be painless; patient response is therefore a poor indicator of uterine action. Contractions may be observed with the hand, recorded with an external tocograph or measured by internal tocography. In normal labour, it is enough to know that the uterus is contracting and that the cervix is dilating. Contractions are crudely quantified in terms of their duration, in seconds, what the observer preceives as mild, moderate or strong, in quality and the frequency of their recurrence. Such observations are recorded on the partogram. Internal tocography provides more exact recording and measurement. This may be particularly important when oxytocin is used in breech presentation, previous caesarean section, grand multiparity or when response to oxytocin is poor (see Chapter 12).

Clinical assessment of fetal size should be attempted and with experience may prove rewarding. The maternal stature is a guide to pelvic size; patients 150 cm tall or less being considered of short stature. Cephalo-pelvic disproportion arises when there is a disparity in fetal and pelvic size sufficient to lead to obstruction. During assessment of a patient in abnormal labour the level of the fetal head above the pelvic brim in fifths is critical. Prior to forceps delivery this is an important observation, and *one fifth* or less should be palpable for this to be safe.

During vaginal examination of the patient in abnormal labour, malpresentation should be excluded and signs of cephalo-pelvic disproportion sought. Failure of the cervix to dilate or the presenting part to descend appropriately, excessive moulding of the head, and palpable restriction of pelvic diameters are all important. Clinical pelvimetry should be performed. Even if inaccurate initially, it is educational to perform, to predict whether disproportion exists and see the result later. *Cephalo-pelvic disproportion* is a retrospective diagnosis made after a well conducted trial of labour fails to bring about flexion, rotation and descent leading to safe vaginal delivery in a patient with a suspect feto-pelvic relationship.

The position of the occiput should be determined during vaginal examination of the patient in abnormal labour. Occipito-posterior position often followed by deflexion of the head is associated with delay in labour. If it does not coexist with disproportion, augmentation of labour is often successful when correct management is undertaken leading to rotation, flexion and descent. This is sometimes referred to as *relative cephalo-pelvic disproportion* (this term has led to confusion and should be discarded). Local cervical problems rarely manifest as cervical dystocia, but previous cervical surgery may be an associated factor. Previously the cervix was often blamed when the power behind it was at fault.

MANAGEMENT OF ABNORMAL LABOUR

Management consists of examination, diagnosis, treatment and review of the unfolding, dynamic process of labour. The active management of labour is a comprehensive management consisting of reassurance, pain relief and oxytocin augmentation of spontaneous labour resulting in limitation of the length of labour and reduction in the number of operative deliveries without detriment to the fetus. Most centres practise augmentation although not the comprehensive approach of O'Driscoll (1986). The approach adopted by Studd is popular. *Augmentation* is ideally instituted if labour progress deviates 2 hours or more to the right of the nomogram on the Studd Stencil (which represents mean progress of normal labour). However, a simple diagonal line drawn at 1 cm per hour from diagnosis of labour, in the active phase, may substitute for the nomogram. Using these criteria, approximately 20% of nulliparae will be augmented, compared to a 50% augmentation rate if the 2 hour allowance is not made.

Whatever the underlying problem, a period of oxytocin augmentation is necessary in most cases before a well conducted trial of labour is complete. Uterine contractions reduce uteroplacental blood flow and continuous electronic fetal heart rate monitoring is desirable, especially when augmentation is prolonged or oxytocin is used in high dosage. Synthetic oxytocin (Syntocinon, Sandoz; Orasthin, Hoechst) is compatible with several types of fluids used for intravenous infusion, but should *not* be given dissolved in 5% dextrose because of the possibility of hyponatraemia. There is also some evidence that it may aggravate fetal acidosis. Normal saline (0.9%) or dextrose saline is most appropriate. The dosage should be calculated in milliunits per minute according to Table 6.2 (see Chapter 6).

Escalation of the tabulated dose at 15 minute intervals permits the optimum dose to be reached in a reasonable period of time by titration against contractions. Contractions should not be more than 5 in every 10 minutes and the uterus should relax adequately between contractions. Such adverse features or abnormal fetal heart rate tracing should prompt temporary cessation or at least reduction of oxytocin dosage. Most patients will respond to less than 12 milliunits per minute, but a difficult induction or a persistent occipito-posterior position may require much more. *Special care should be taken to exclude mechanical obstruction in the multiparous patient. Intrauterine pressure measurement is desirable in difficult cases.* Poorly controlled oxytocin infusions are associated with fetal distress, and a peristaltic infusion drip counter should be used. High doses of oxytocin have been associated with hyponatraemia and neonatal hyperbilirubinaemia.

Assessment of the response to augmentation should be made at two-hourly intervals and signs of obstruction sought, namely; arrest of dilatation and descent of the presenting part, excessive moulding, and restriction of pelvic diameters. Taking into account fetal and maternal condition, a decision about whether to continue to strive for vaginal delivery should be made.

Using this method of assessment, failure to progress in labour ceases to be an indication for caesarean section without further specification of the underlying cause. The operation note should always confirm the position, head level and presence or absence of moulding at caesarean section. The picture may be completed by postpartum radiological pelvimetry, and such information used in planning future deliveries. Early diagnosis, appropriate augmentation and two-hourly review results in fetus and mother remaining in optimal condition and permits a decision to be made on the mode of delivery before excessive prolongation of labour occurs.

6

Intravenous Fluid Management

Pregnancy is a physiological state experienced by fit young women with normal metabolism and normal renal function. Fluid management in abnormal states is therefore not considered here. Pregnancy has been described as an accelerated starvation syndrome. A pregnant woman starved for caesarean section almost always develops ketonuria, whereas a non-pregnant woman similarly starved for hysterectomy rarely does. It is important that this situation should not be compounded unwittingly in labour.

Low-risk patients in early labour may suck ice cubes or have small amounts of glucose drinks. In complicated labour this is undesirable because delayed gastric emptying, characteristic of pregnancy, increases the risk of aspiration of stomach contents should anaesthesia become necessary. Prior to induction of labour by artificial rupture of the membranes, breakfast should be omitted on the morning of the procedure. If prostaglandin induction is planned, there is no objection to an early breakfast and further oral intake if labour does not become established quickly. Compounding prolonged starvation with prolonged induction of labour is undesirable.

Women who have short, efficient labours do not require intravenous fluids; the siting of a cannula is unnecessary and intrusive. When intravenous fluids are required during labour, a large forearm vein should be selected, a cannula of at least 16-gauge with a side-arm inserted and a long giving set used to permit easy access, concurrent infusions and mobility.

Intravenous fluids are given during labour for:
1 Hydration
2 As a vehicle for drugs
3 Provision of energy, as calories
4 In the diabetic patient
5 In association with epidural anaesthesia
6 Special situations
   Blood transfusion other than in the management of haemorrhage

is undesirable because it further complicates a potentially hazardous situation.

Hydration

Women are more likely to become dehydrated than overhydrated in labour. Most labouring women are fit and young with normal renal function and the normal daily requirement of 3 litres is increased because of physical exertion, sweating and increased metabolism. Dehydration in the later stages of labour may manifest itself as reduced urinary output and a steadily rising fetal heart rate resulting in a tachycardia. This can be reversed by an infusion of normal saline or Hartmann's solution. A standard intravenous giving set delivers 1 ml as 20 drops. Table 6.1 shows equivalent volumes at various rates.

Table 6.1 Drop rate–volume conversion.

Drops per min	Volume per min (ml)	Volume per 12 h (ml)	Volume per 24 h (ml)
10	0.5	360	720
20	1.0	720	1440
30	1.5	1080	2160
40	2.0	1440	2880
50	2.5	1800	3600
60	3.0	2160	4320

It is seen that at 30 drops per minute, about 1 litre is delivered in 12 hours; at 60 drops per minute this is just over 2 litres. Normal saline or Hartmann's solution is physiological and should be used for hydration. Dextrose saline may be used when an element of caloric intake is desirable. Pure dextrose solution, especially concentrated, should be avoided because of potential precipitation of electrolyte imbalance or fetal distress.

A vehicle for drugs

The drug most commonly used during labour is synthetic oxytocin (Syntocinon, Sandoz; Orasthin, Hoechst). This can be given in a concentrated form from a syringe pump. However, a gravity-fed

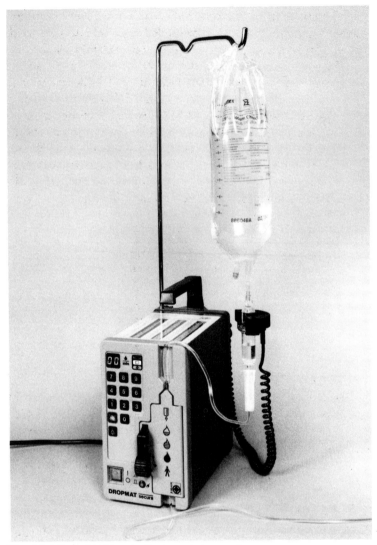

Fig. 6.1. *Peristaltic drip controller.*

infusion (a drip) is convenient and adequate. An infusion solution containing oxytocin should not be used during insertion of the cannula into the vein because a bolus of oxytocin may be inadvertently administered, resulting in uterine hypertonus. After the cannula has been sited using saline, the oxytocin should be administered in 1 litre of normal saline through the side arm. The infusion bag used for setting up may then be used at a variable rate to adjust hydration. The oxytocin infusion should be controlled using an unsophisticated peristaltic drip controller (Fig. 6.1). More complex infusion pumps, especially volumetric ones using disposable cassette systems, are expensive and unnecessary. Oxytocin is a drug and its dosage should be monitored. Inadequate dosage will fail to correct poor uterine action whilst excessive dosage may lead to hypertonic uterine contractions, abnormal fetal heart rate patterns, uterine rupture, hyperbilirubinaemia in the neonate, and electrolyte imbalance in the labouring woman. Table 6.2 shows a method for calculating oxytocin dosage. Comparison of Tables 6.1 and 6.2 shows that using the concentrations shown, overhydration should not occur.

Table 6.2 Oxytocin dose calculation (milliunits per minute).

Drops per min	4 units per litre	8 units per litre	16 units per litre	32 units per litre
10	2	4	8	16
20	4	8	16	32
30	6	12	24	48
40	8	16	32	64
50	10	20	40	80
60	12	24	48	96

Other regimens of oxytocin infusion may be used, bearing in mind concentration–dose conversions. However, uniformity of method leads to better understanding and communication between staff. The interval at which the drip rate should be increased is discussed in the chapter on the treatment of abnormal labour progress.

Energy provision

Mobilization of glycogen stores and fatty acids provides a supply of energy in the fasting patient. Ketosis in labour is a manifestation of the pregnant stage and possibly of dehydration. Rehydration, irrespective of energy supply, will often correct it. Some years ago, there was a tendency to give 10%, 30% or 50% glucose to 'fortify' patients. Such treatment is unphysiological and potentially hazardous. It may result in maternal and neonatal hyponatraemia, lactic acidosis and neonatal hypoglycaemia. 5% and 10% glucose infusions have also been implicated as possible causes of neonatal jaundice. Maintenance of physiological levels of blood sugar achieved by infusion of 5% dextrose or 4% dextrose saline at ɔɔ drops per minute as in the diabetic patient in labour (50 g dextrose over 12 hours).

Diabetes mellitus

The principle of therapy in the diabetic patient in labour is to maintain tight glucose homeostasis by concomitant infusion of insulin and 5% dextrose governed by regular, frequent blood glucose estimation. This is done using a glucometer and based on a regimen where 1 unit of insulin per hour is infused intravenously to interact with approximately 5 g of dextrose per hour (100 ml of 5% dextrose). Oxytocin or any other therapy has to be given through another infusion. Further discussion of the diabetic patient is beyound the scope of this book.

Epidural anaesthesia

Effective epidural anaesthesia abolishes the sympathetic tone of the peripheral vasculature. There is consequent vasodilatation and pooling of circulating blood volume in the peripheral tissues. This may result in hypotension, defective uteroplacental perfusion, and an abnormal fetal heart rate pattern. Blood pressure and heart rate monitoring are always undertaken in the patient with an epidural. These adverse effects can be anticipated and avoided by preloading with 500–1000 ml of Hartmann's solution prior to epidural siting.

Special situations

Inhibition of labour using a beta-sympathomimetic drug combined with steroid therapy to induce lung maturity is hazardous unless great care is taken with intravenous fluids. This may be further compromised by the greatly increased circulating volume in normal pregnancy. Fluids should be isotonic and limited in volume; meticulous fluid balance is essential.

The use of very high dose oxytocin dissolved in hypotonic fluids infused over a long period is undesirable because of the risk of hyponatraemia. This situation may arise in second-trimester abortion or management of hydatidiform mole; other therapy is more appropriate.

7

Pain Relief

Pain is subjective. Some women find childbirth extremely painful, whilst others experience only mild discomfort. Good preparation through antenatal classes will reduce anxiety, educate and otherwise prepare the pregnant woman. Knowing the person who is going to look after her also helps, but unfortunately the chances of meeting a pre-arranged carer in labour are small, bearing in mind current conditions in government-funded hospitals. Caroline Flint (1986) has published a report on an example of a 'Know your Midwife' scheme. Emotionally, continuity of care in such a scheme must be highly desirable; remaining obstacles are financial and organisational. Nonetheless, a good relationship between a woman and her carer in labour is indispensible. Currently, the use of pharmacological methods of pain relief in labour is declining. Psychoprophylaxis is important and there is increasing interest in transcutaneous nerve stimulation (TENS). Increasingly women are finding that no analgesia or inhalational analgesia are adequate. Homeopathy, acupuncture and hypnosis may have a role to play, and back massage and diversion of attention by a repetitive act such as clicking the fingers are found useful by many.

INHALATIONAL METHOD

The only inhalational method remaining is Entonox. Trilene and Penthrane are no longer approved for use by the United Kingdom Central Council (UKCC) of midwives. Entonox should only be used for a limited time late in labour.
- Entonox is a 50 : 50 mixture of nitrous oxide and oxygen. When stored at a low temperature, the gases separate, and so the cylinder must warm up to room temperature.
- Contractions in the late first stage and second stage are generally regular. The woman must anticipate a contraction and start breathing 30 seconds before the contraction begins. She then stops inhaling

during the contraction and can concentrate on the expulsive effort
as appropriate.

● Long deep breaths triggering the inhalational valve are best. The
woman should hold the mask and control the inhalation herself.

● Gasping and rapid inspiration may lead to tetany due to metabolic
alkalosis.

● Excessive use leads to drowsiness and confusion. Controlled use
is essential. There are no serious adverse effects.

PARENTERAL OPIATES

Intramuscular pethidine

● It is given in a dosage of 50–150 mg depending on the degree
of pain, body weight and other factors.

● It is routinely given intramuscularly, often combined with Phenergan to control nausea and augment the effect. In fact, many women
are not nauseated and the effect of Phenergan on the fetus is not
clear. It may therefore be better to administer pethidine alone and
give metoclopramide if nausea and vomiting are troublesome.

● It may be given in repeated dosage. Some are hesitant to give it
near the end of the first stage of labour. However, it does not always
depress the neonate seriously and this effect can easily be managed
by the paediatrician.

● Pethidine is disliked by some women because it induces a state
of drowsiness and confusion. Memories of such labours are not
pleasant.

Intravenous pethidine or diamorphine

● Pethidine, 75 mg, or diamorphine, 5 mg, may be given intravenously in an acute situation. This induces immediate relaxation.

● If a patient is particularly restless or distressed when assisted delivery is necessary and urgent, this is the method of choice. It has a
particular place in shoulder dystocia. To struggle in such a situation
with the patient unable to co-operate is very difficult. Administration
of general anaesthesia takes time and is an unwarranted additional
risk. In such a situation, the anaesthetist is likely to be present anyway
and can manage any respiratory difficulty possibly occurring after
intravenous opiates.

- This treatment also represents an alternative to the routine use of epidural in breech and twin delivery. Preservation of the expulsive sensation and effort is a great advantage. An anaesthetist standing by for these cases is very important.

EPIDURAL ANALGESIA

- This is a very effective method of pain relief in labour and is especially appropriate for elective caesarean section. Several practical points require consideration, and careful management is important. Provision of a 24 hour epidural service is desirable. However, women should be discouraged from deciding to have an epidural prior to the start of labour. They should be reassured that a full armamentarium of methods of pain relief is available. The decision should be made during labour, bearing in mind the clinical situation. Nulliparous, anxious patients experiencing a lot of pain in early labour are the obvious candidates, especially if an occipito-posterior position is suspected or a mechanical problem anticipated.
- Coagulopathy is a *contraindication* to epidural analgesia. In most pre-eclamptics the coagulation profile is normal. However, it should be checked first. Lumbar skin sepsis, disease of the spine and neurological disorders are *relative* contraindications.
- An intravenous infusion must be set up prior to the siting of the epidural. Hypotension may occur due to peripheral vasodilatation. This should be anticipated and avoided by giving 1 litre of Hartmann's solution whilst preparing for the anaesthetist. Hypotension and concomitant abnormality of the fetal heart rate may be avoided by this manoeuvre.
- Although the earlier part of labour is unaffected, epidural analgesia is associated with delay in the late first stage and second stage. By virtue of the woman having been selected for epidural, this may have been destined to happen anyway. There are several possible mechanisms, but absence of the urge to push and secondary uterine inertia play a part. This can be counteracted by delaying topping-up, half dose topping-up, topping-up whilst seated upright, and active use of oxytocin for failure of descent. The criteria for use of oxytocin in the second stage for augmentation are more subtle than in the first stage, but just as important.
- Active pushing should be discouraged until the presenting part is visible on separating the labia.

- Women appreciate having effective pain relief in the first stage of labour but are also motivated to have an unassisted delivery.
- Epidural top-up is very useful prior to repair of genital tract lacerations, episiotomy, exploration of the uterus and manual removal of the placenta.

CAUDAL ANALGESIA

- A one-shot caudal analgesia is useful if the patient, who requires mid-cavity or rotational forceps delivery, has not had epidural prior to this situation arising.

GENERAL ANAESTHESIA

- This should rarely be necessary to effect vaginal delivery and substantially increases the risk to the mother, especially under emergency circumstances. If it is given then, halothane should be avoided because of its utero-relaxant properties and the possibility of postpartum haemorrhage. It is sometimes seen as an easy option when maternal discomfort is severe and co-operation limited. Intravenous opiates are an alternative. As well as the increased risks of general anaesthesia, depriving a couple of seeing their child being born is undesirable.
- Every opportunity should be taken to give ranitidine, 150 mg intravenously, and sodium citrate before general anaesthesia in the obstetric patient. The application of cricoid pressure is also mandatory to reduce the risk of inhalation of gastric contents.
- A policy for the prevention of Mendelson's syndrome (aspiration of gastric contents) should be formulated. An H_2-receptor antagonist such as ranitidine given to labouring women at risk of operative delivery appears effective.

8

Pre-term and Post-term Labour

Ninety percent of women deliver at term; between 37 completed weeks of gestation and 42 completed weeks of gestation. About 7% deliver *pre-term* and 3% deliver *post-term*. *Premature membrane rupture* is membrane rupture occurring before the onset of labour, irrespective of gestation. A *low birth weight* baby weighs less than 2500 g. Most pre-term babies are of low birth weight although not all low birth weight babies are pre-term: they may be small for dates. A *very low birth weight* baby weighs less than 1500 g.

PRE-TERM LABOUR

Predisposing factors

- Previous pre-term delivery
- Young age
- Poor social class

Associated clinical features

- Polyhydramnios
- Multiple gestation
- Antepartum haemorrhage
- Cervical incompetence, uterine abnormality
- Membrane rupture

If there are no associated features it is termed uncomplicated pre-term labour.

Diagnosis

This rests on the same principles as the diagnosis of labour at term. If the presenting part is high, contractions irregular, and the cervix uneffaced, the diagnosis is improbable. In many studies of the use of beta-mimetic drugs in pre-term labour there have been a large number of placebo responses, the likely explanation of which is that many of the cases were not in pre-term labour. Ultrasound may have a role to play in resolving this dilemma. In the absence of multiple pregnancy, rupture of the membranes, and antepartum haemorrhage, the presence of fetal breathing makes delivery within 48 hours unlikely. Ultrasound is also useful in the management of the woman at risk of pre-term delivery, to determine fetal weight and presentation and to exclude major malformations (see Chapter 15).

Management: inhibition of labour

The management will depend on neonatal intensive care facilities available and the possibility of *in utero* transfer to a referral centre.
• Consider transfer. Beta-mimetics, if indicated, during transfer
• Gestation > 32 weeks; monitor FH continuously; proceed to delivery
• Gestation < 32 weeks; consider beta-mimetics for 48 hours to allow for dexamethasone to be given; monitor fetal heart when contracting, and twice daily

Beta-mimetic drugs: Ritodrine, salbutamol, fenoterol, isoxuprine, orciprenaline and terbutaline. Which drug is used, and whether it is used depends on availability in different countries and local habit. Some centres and countries do not use beta-mimetics or steriods at all for pre-term labour.

Dose of Ritodrine: 50 μg/min, increasing by 50 μg/min every 10 minutes until maternal heart rate is greater than 120. Effective dose usually 150–350 μg/min.

Beta-mimetics are relatively contraindicated in:
• Pre-existing cardiac disease
• Antepartum haemorrhage
• Diabetes mellitus (due to hyperglycaemic effect)
• Chorioamnionitis
• Other conditions of hostile intrauterine environment
Side effects include palpitations, chest discomfort, sweating and tremor. Patients do not feel comfortable on a therapeutic dose. Chest pain or dyspnoea during treatment should lead to immediate cessation of therapy. Myocardial ischaemia and cardiac failure have been reported particularly when a combination of large volumes of in-

travenous fluids, steroids and sympathomimetics have been used. Beta-mimetic infusion should be discontinued 6 hours after cessation of contractions. There is little evidence that oral therapy is useful unless maternal tachycardia and side effects are induced. There is no doubt that a bolus infusion of a beta-mimetic drug stops the uterus contracting, but there is little evidence that beta-mimetics generally reduce the incidence of pre-term labour or influence the outcome. When it is necessary to use beta-mimetics on several occasions over a few days, worthwhile prolongation of the pregnancy is unlikely. Greater awareness of potentially serious side effects has limited their use in recent years. The principle value of beta-mimetics may be in the time gained in order to give dexamethasone or to organise *in utero* transfer.

Management: acute use of beta-mimetics

They may have a place in the immediate management of fetal distress due to uterine hypertonus or cord compression. A bolus dose of 200 μg of terbutaline results in cessation of uterine contractions for at least 30 minutes.

Dexamethasone (24 mg in divided doses) has been shown to reduce the incidence of hyaline membrane disease in the neonate when given between 28 and 32 weeks' gestation. There is no statistically significant reduction in hyaline membrane disease after 32 weeks and it has not been studied before 28 weeks. Some authorities have not been convinced by its effects and its use is variable.

The combination of dexamethasone and beta-mimetics appears to increase the probability of cardiovascular side effects in the mother. Large volumes of intravenous fluids are also hazardous.

Management: mode of delivery

Considerable controversy surrounds the question of how these babies, especially those of less than 1500 g, should be delivered. There has been a tendency, particularly when the presentation is breech, to deliver by caesarean section. This appears logical when it is a footling breech with a high risk of umbilical and prolapse and entrapment of the aftercoming head. Although retrospective analyses have reached differing conclusions, there has been no randomized,

prospective, controlled trial. If caesarean section is performed then
it should be planned carefully. After opening the abdomen, the uterus
should be inspected to determine the type of uterine incision which
will lead to least traumatic delivery of the baby. The investment of
careful assessment of the high risk pregnancy should not be squan-
dered by difficult extraction of the baby through an inadequate
uterine incision.

Pre-term vaginal delivery

There is no evidence that forceps protect the pre-term baby's head
from trauma. A large episiotomy, if the perineum is resistant in any
way, and delivery by a skilled person are usually satisfactory. Obstetric
and paediatric staff should be present.

Premature membrane rupture (PROM)

This is membrane rupture occurring before the onset of labour,
irrespective of gestation. The implications of this carry a greater risk
to the fetus when it occurs very early in gestation; pre-term premature
membrane rupture (PPROM).

Always perform speculum examination to confirm the diagnosis;
never perform digital examination if conservative management is an
option. Cord compression is diagnosed from the fetal heart rate
tracing *not* digital examination.
- < 32 weeks: Vaginal swabs for microbiology. Consider amniocentesis to exclude infection and detailed ultrasound, including amniotic fluid volume assessment. Steroids and beta-mimetic cover if
no infection. Planned delivery when natural onset.
- > 32 weeks: Vaginal swab for microbiology. Wait 48 hours if
no signs of infection. Use oxytocin stimulation if prognosis for labour
good. Perform amniocentesis if option to conserve pregnancy.

The challenge is to balance the risks of infection on the one hand
against risks of prematurity on the other. The concern is that
chorioamnionitis may precede PROM. It does not usually follow,
unless digital examinations have been done unwisely. If infection has
preceded PROM, labour may well follow. Bearing this in mind,
amniocentesis to exclude infection is most appropriate in the first 48
hours after PROM. The signs of chorioamnionitis appear late:
- Pyrexia

- Tachycardia
- Lower uterine tenderness
- Change in the nature of vaginal discharge especially if foul smelling

With evidence of established infection, caesarean section is the mode of delivery. Operating on a grossly infected organ (as occurs in developing countries) is undesirable, but that is not the situation here.

POST-TERM (POSTMATURE) LABOUR

Whether it is spontaneous or induced, labour after 42 weeks of gestation constitutes a high risk. In such cases the menstrual, clinical and ultrasound dating history should be carefully reviewed.

- Meconium staining of the amniotic fluid is more frequent whether due to maturity or asphyxia.
- Continuous intrapartum fetal heart rate monitoring should be performed.
- Consideration taken of the possibility that a high level of the presenting part with a big baby in the first pregnancy is the aetiology. This has serious implications for the trial of labour.
- Prolongation of the second stage is undesirable when postmaturity, meconium staining of the amniotic fluid and decelerations are present.

A baby resulting from a postmature pregnancy should be checked thoroughly by the paediatrician. Evidence of the postmaturity syndrome in the neonate is important, however, this only manifests in a very small minority of cases.

9

Induction of Labour

Labour is induced when there is evidence that continuation of the pregnancy entails greater risk to the mother and/or the fetus than delivery. This may pertain in many conditions, but interpretation in different centres leads to induction rates varying from 3% to 35%. The 1980s have seen a decline in induction for several reasons. The use and reliability of tests of fetal well-being have been important, as well as differing local conditions and changing attitudes.

Several methods of induction are effective, but labour should be induced in the labour ward, in daytime and with full fetal monitoring facilities. Methods of induction were previously referred to as medical or surgical, but the distinction has become blurred and these terms should be rejected. In selecting the method of induction the concept of the *readiness* of that uterus for labour should be considered. It is not only the cervix that is ripe (see Chapter 10), but the whole organ. The uterus in mid-pregnancy is not ready for labour, oxytocin receptors not yet having developed. On the other hand the uterus that has threatened pre-term labour, from which there has been bleeding or which has displayed irritability with many Braxton–Hicks contractions is readier. The evidence for readiness is accessible in the cervix (see Table 1.1); if the cervical score is 6 or more, it is favourable.

Methods:
- Oxytocin infusion alone
- Artificial rupture of the membranes (ARM)
- ARM and oxytocin
- Prostaglandins locally *per vaginam*
- Other routes of prostaglandin administration (see Chapter 10)

Oxytocin infusion alone

This is ineffective well before term unless the membranes have already ruptured (PROM—see below). Oxytocin has been used to prime the cervix prior to ARM; however, there are risks. In the presence

44

of a favourable cervix it is better to rupture the membranes to examine the colour of the amniotic fluid. If oxytocin is given with intact membranes, and then the membranes rupture or are ruptured artificially, there is a cumulative effect on uterine contractility and hyperstimulation may occur. There is the added rare, but lethal risk of amnotic fluid embolism which has been documented under these circumstances.

ARM alone

This is performed with Kocher's forceps or an Amnihook. Lithotomy position and extensive sterile precautions are unnecessary. It is preferably done with the head at least settling into the pelvic brim (3/5 palpable), and an assistant may apply abdominal pressure. Mild analgesia may be indicated. The colour of the amniotic fluid is examined, cord prolapse sought digitally, and monitoring commenced immediately. A proportion of patients will not go into labour even within 24 hours and it is better to follow ARM with an oxytocin infusion. The place for ARM alone is in the woman, usually multiparous, with a favourable cervix who has expressed a desire for a natural birth, but who has accepted induction. An intravenous infusion may be avoided under these circumstances. The same result may be achieved using prostaglandin pessaries.

ARM and oxytocin infusion

This combination has stood the test of time as the safest method of induction when the cervix is favourable. It is gentle to the fetus, but effective. After ARM, 30 minutes of fetal heart rate tracing is performed to check fetal condition before the added stress of oxytocin. Oxytocin is then commenced and escalated in the same regimen as for augmentation (see Chapter 5). Once the cervix is 5 cm dilated the dose can be reduced substantially (by at least 60%) and labour maintained. If this reduction is not done, hyperstimulation may occur. Vaginal examination is performed every 2–3 hours.

Prostaglandins

Enthusiasm for prostaglandin induction has been tempered by the recognition of uterine hyperstimulation in cases with a favourable cervix. Nonetheless, prostaglandins are potent oxytocics and have a role to play in the woman with an unfavourable cervix (cervical score 5 or less). They are effective when given systemically, but side effects are a problem. Vaginal administration is the route of choice and PGE_2 (3 mg) pessaries (Prostin E_2, Upjohn) are most readily available.

There are two regimens of administration but whichever is chosen, fetal condition must be carefully checked. One method aims to induce and deliver whilst the other attempts ripening over a more prolonged period. It is acknowledged that induction should not be a very prolonged procedure.

1 Restricting prostaglandin induction to cases with an unfavourable cervix, one pessary (3 mg) is given at 8 a.m. The patient remains recumbent and monitored for the first hour. If contractions do not supervene, she may mobilize. At 1 p.m., another vaginal examination is performed. If labour has not started and the cervix is unchanged, another pessary is given and further monitoring undertaken. In diabetic and other high-risk patients, an ARM is always attempted rather than giving a second pessary. All patients proceed to ARM and oxytocin if necessary by late afternoon. This ensures delivery by late evening by whatever method which seems a reasonable physical and psychological proposition. Further repetition of pessary administration usually proves fruitless and is not advised. ARM should not be performed shortly after a pessary has been given because the cumulative effect of endogenous and exogenous prostaglandin is undesirable.

2 Prostaglandins are also used for 'slow' inductions where it is thought the effect takes up to 24 hours to be seen. This is also referred to as cervical priming. It is impossible to predict prospectively which cases will be primed and which induced—in fact the process is the same, only progressing at a different speed. In 'slow' induction, a pessary is inserted one morning, the patient initially being monitored. If labour does not begin, the same process is repeated the following morning, then followed later that day by ARM. If a woman needs induction, she needs delivery and it is undesirable that such a procedure should continue for several days. This is especially true in the hypertensive patient. Special caution should be exercised in giving prostaglandin pessaries in the evening to unmonitored patients. By definition these patients must be at risk because they are being induced. The hours of darkness are not the optimum time for delivery.

Other routes of prostaglandin administration

Several parenteral methods have been used successfully, however, the incidence of side effects is higher.

STIMULATION OF LABOUR

This is referred to by many people as induction of labour. However, by common usage it has come to mean the use of oxytocics in the patient with premature rupture of the membranes (PROM). Premature rupture of the membranes is loss of amniotic fluid without the concomitant onset of labour. It may occur at any gestation, but when it occurs before term and especially much earlier in pregnancy (PPROM) it carries a greater risk to the fetus (see Chapter 8).

Diagnosis

The diagnosis must be confirmed by speculum examination, visualization of fluid, or the use of Amnistix. Digital examinations must *not* be performed because of the increased risk of infection, unless delivery has already been planned in the near future. Cord compression is excluded by a normal fetal heart rate tracing.

Management

At term it is probably safe to wait at least 24 hours, during which time more than half the cases will go into spontaneous labour, as long as the patient is showing no signs of infection. When delivery is indicated, the cervix can be digitally assessed and appropriate stimulation given depending on favourability. This can be by oxytocin infusion or prostaglandin pessaries.

Monitoring in induced and stimulated labour

Uterine contractions, especially when iatrogenic, stress the fetus. The fetus must already be considered to be at some risk in this situation and careful heart rate monitoring is mandatory. The contractions must also be monitored carefully in an attempt to produce contractions which mimic normal labour.

10

Mid-trimester Termination of Pregnancy

Emptying the uterus poses more of a problem in mid-pregnancy than towards term. The myometrium and cervix are unprimed, requiring the use of prostaglandins which are very effective in this situation.

This section concerns the termination of wanted pregnancy in which some unfortunate event, such as intrauterine death or detection of a fetal anomaly has occurred. Termination of pregnancy is legal in the United Kingdom until 28 weeks of gestation. This is currently under review at the time of writing. However, most specialists will only undertake it after 20 weeks of gestation for the indications considered here. Such women deserve special management, close relationships with staff, effective analgesia and constant vigilance to minimize sequelae especially of a psychological nature. Ideally, there should be a small area set aside for such cases between obstetric and gynaecological services (see Chapter 24).

DILATATION AND EVACUATION

A few specialists will perform this in the mid-trimester but it should only be done by those with great experience. General anaesthesia is used; it is quicker and may be kinder to the patient. Cervical damage, uterine damage, retained products of conception and haemorrhage are important risks. Real-time ultrasound has a place in ensuring complete emptying of the uterus. The disadvantage is that pathological examination of the fetus is difficult. This is desirable, especially for confirmation of fetal malformation.

PROSTAGLANDINS

Most practitioners will perform termination of pregnancy by the vacuum aspiration method in the first trimester of pregnancy (Fig. 10.1). Vaginal pessaries in the form of gemeprost (Cervagem) have a role to play in softening and dilating the nulliparous cervix when given 3 hours prior to instrumental dilatation. There are various possible roles of prostaglandins in the management of second trimester termination of pregnancy.

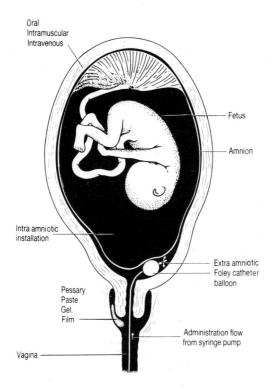

Fig. 10.1. *Routes of prostaglandin administration.*

Prior to 18 weeks gestation

Gemeprost (Cervagem), which has recently become more freely available, is effective when given as a 1 mg pessary every 3 hours, about five times. Its effect can be augmented with oxytocin infusion at the end of this 15 hour period, or when the membranes rupture. However, it is not yet licensed for this purpose and extra-amniotic infusion still has a place.

Extra-amniotic

Prior to this procedure, nervous patients should be given sedation because insertion of the catheter may be painful. A Foley catheter is passed through the cervix, and the bag inflated with 30 ml of sterile water. Maximal inflation is important (so that the balloon does not fall out) until the cervix is at least 3 cm dilated. Prostaglandin, at 1 ml per hour, is infused through the catheter maintained by a syringe pump. Lack of uterine response suggests the need to increase the dose which may be up to 6 ml per hour. Care must be taken to fill the dead space in the catheter, ensure integrity of the system and check the pump is working. Technical problems in maintaining the system functional make this a troublesome and imperfect method. The disadvantage in late termination of malformed fetuses by this method is that the fetus is often born with a heart beat, possibly moving and breathing. This is psychologically traumatic for the couple and the staff. Intra-amniotic methods obviate this difficulty and should be used after 18 weeks.

After 18 weeks; intra-amniotic

The patient is sedated and amniocentesis done under ultrasound guidance. A small amount of fluid is removed (this may be sent for chromosomal analysis) and prostaglandin E_2, 5 mg with 10 mg of urea, is injected. Hypertonic saline increases the risk of this method. The needle is then removed. Patience is required and contractions start in most cases by twelve hours. If this does not occur the addition of gemeprost pessaries or an extra-amniotic approach usually proves effective.

Although the WHO have conducted studies of intramuscular prostaglandins for this purpose they are not available.

11

Fetal Well-being—Heart Rate Monitoring

How is the fetus? This question must be asked, taking into account fetal condition over the preceding weeks leading up to today, the day of delivery; the most dangerous journey to be undertaken. The starting point of the assessment of fetal wellbeing is basic clinical observation. Admission to the labour ward is a good time for review.

The following risk factors are especially important in the *history*:

- Prematurity or postmaturity
- Poor fetal growth
- Vaginal bleeding
- Hypertension, diabetes, medical conditions
- Breech presentation, multiple pregnancy
- Reduced fetal movements
  On abdominal examination, emphasis is placed on:
- Symphysis fundal height
- Fetal presentation, station and size
- Amniotic fluid volume
- Amniotic fluid colour if ROM
- Contractions

The fetal heart should be auscultated, the rate recorded and an admission cardiotcograph (CTG) performed on all patients and reported as follows:

- Technical quality
- Baseline rate
- Baseline variability
- Periodic changes:
  accelerations
  decelerations, nature
- Contractions

A well grown fetus, with normal movements, normal amniotic fluid, no risk factors and a normal admission CTG is unlikely to die in the following few hours unless subject to placental abruption or

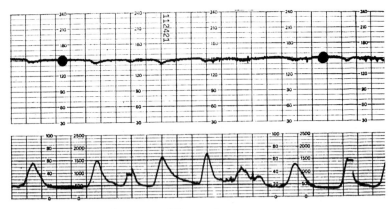

Fig. 11.1. *Ominous flat trace; audibly normal.*

umbilical cord prolapse; such events should be detected with clinical skill.

There is no such thing as 'no-risk', only 'low-risk' and 'high-risk'. Women with risk factors (as above) should be monitored continuously. The admission trace is crucial. Fig. 11.1 shows an admission trace of a fetal heart, recorded in a study without information being given to the clinician, which was auscultated and reported as normal at the dots. The fetus was in the preterminal stages of asphyxia. Auscultation tells us nothing about baseline variability. The absence of this is the most crucial feature of this trace. High-risk fetuses should be monitored continuously by electronic means. Flexibility complementing clinical monitoring with electronic monitoring is realistic in other cases.

CLINICAL MONITORING

Auscultation of the fetal heart with a Pinard stethoscope should be performed regularly and appropriately. The alternative to continuous electronic monitoring is not 'no monitoring' but careful, intelligent, clinical monitoring. Eletronic monitoring can be used to supplement this intermittently. Auscultation involves sampling only a tiny interval, but, if done every 15 minutes in the first stage just after a contraction, and after every contraction in the late first stage and second stage, may pick up significant abnormalities. Shortage of paper and machines sharpens clinical acumen! They are best used for high-risk patients, admission traces, and traces in late labour if there is a shortage of equipment.

Meconium is the fetal intestinal contents. It is passed into the amniotic fluid for two reasons; because of advancing maturity and because of fetal compromise. Meconium staining of the amniotic fluid is uncommon before 35 weeks gestation. However, it is seen in 15% of pregnancies at 42 weeks. It is generally thin and old under these circumstances, being passed with advancing maturation of the gastrointestinal tract. Although steps should be taken to guard against inspiration by the fetus it is usually innocuous as long as the fetal heart rate is normal. Fresh meconium is passed by some fetuses which are actuely *compromised*. In *uncompromised* breech presentation it is passed directly through the cervix as the fetal abdomen is compressed with descent of the breech. In cephalic presentation, it is the fresh appearance of meconium or a change in its nature during labour that is so important. Meconium can only be thick and fresh ('pea soup') in cephalic presentation if there is *oligohydramnios* with no dilution; this means *compromise*. Amniotic fluid should be sought during vaginal examination by pushing the head gently upwards if there is any doubt about fetal well-being and amniotic fluid is not draining spontaneously.

Meconium aspiration syndrome causes serious morbidity in babies near term. It may occur *in utero* or during delivery itself. A fetus will gasp *in utero* when it is distressed, with an abnormal fetal heart rate pattern. This results in lodging of sticky meconium in the terminal bronchioles. Unless labour is short and efficient, caesarean section should be expedited in a case with thick meconium and an abnormal tracing. During vaginal delivery in patients with meconium staining of the amniotic fluid, a paediatrician should always be in attendance. Aspiration of the oropharynx (*not* the nose which stimulates gasping) should be done after the head is delivered. Splinting of the chest is not useful but, after delivery, the vocal cords should be visualised and material aspirated.

Blood staining of the amniotic fluid is an important sign (see Chapter 18). It should be distinguished from blood arising from the mucus plug and cervix after digital examination which results in non-uniform staining.

PHYSIOLOGY OF FETAL HEART CONTROL

The interpretation of fetal heart rate traces is facilitated by an understanding of the mechanism controlling cardiac activity. The sino-atrial node has an intrinsic rate which is modulated by the autonomic nervous system. The sympathetic system increases the heart rate whilst the parasympathetic lowers it; the former acting more slowly than the latter. The continuous interplay between the elevation of heart rate by sympathetic stimulation and lowering by parasympathetic stimulation results in a beat-to-beat fluctuation in rate which is known as *variability*. Sympathetic response develops quite early in fetal life, whereas parasympathetic response does not become pronounced until later in pregnancy. The preterm fetus therefore may show a higher baseline fetal heart rate with less variability. The key to understanding asphyxial features on a trace is the evidence of integrity of autonomic control, and this is progressively lost as asphyxia becomes more serious. Baseline rate, baseline variability and features before and after decelerations are crucial.

ELECTRONIC FETAL HEART RATE MONITORING

This may be performed by the following techniques (Fig. 11.2):
1 External ultrasound
2 Internal fetal scalp electrode

The second method generally produces a better quality tracing. However, modern equipment using autocorrelation techniques produce improved, cleaner external traces. Patients wishing to remain mobile will be better monitored with an electrode than externally. Telemetry may be useful, particularly for women with risk factors wishing to remain mobile.

TRACE ANALYSIS

Duration: In the United Kingdom the normal paper speed is 1 cm per minute, whilst in the United States of America it is 3 cm per minute. This must be borne in mind when evaluating duration and baseline variability. At 1 cm per minute the length of a segment of major division (between bold lines) is 10 minutes.

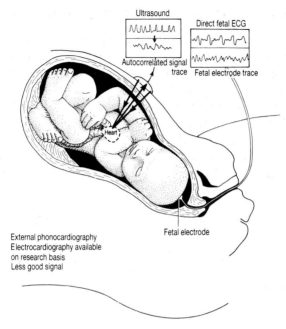

Fig. 11.2. *Modes of fetal heart rate monitoring.*

Technical quality: This may be so bad as to be uninterpretable and steps should be taken to improve it. If quality is very poor then effectively these patients should be regarded as unmonitored electronically, and intermittent auscultation performed. This may become very relevant in cases where litigation has ensued. Bad data may be worse than no data.

Baseline rate: Baseline rate is identified when periods of acceleration and deceleration are excluded. The normal rate is 110 to 150 beats per minute (b.p.m.). A baseline rate of 150 b.p.m. is likely to be rising to a pathological tachycardia whereas a rate of 110 b.p.m. is more often stable. It is not uncommon to see a baseline rate of 110 b.p.m., good variability, reactivity and excellent outcome (Fig. 11.3). Further reference should be made to the report of FIGO Subcommittee on Standards in Perinatal Medicine (1987).

Baseline variability: This is the feature that causes greatest confusion. It is not the same as beat-to-beat variability, which is not discernable and generally not specifically measured by most machines, which

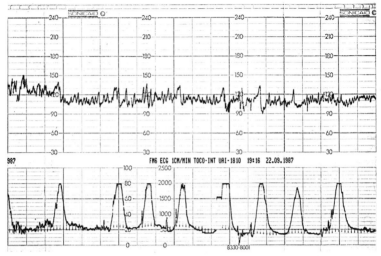

Fig. 11.3. *Low baseline; reactive.*

depend on a technique of averaging several beat intervals. It is important, being clearly related to asphyxia. Although oscillatory frequency
and amplitude are the keys to interpretation this is simplified by the
concept of band width. A segment of baseline tracing should be
examined and its band width determined (Fig. 11.4). A band width
of 10–25 b.p.m. is normal, 5–10 b.p.m. is reduced, less than 5
b.p.m. is a silent pattern, and greater than 25 b.p.m. is saltatory.
The vertical scale in beats per minute must be considered when
evaluating variability. Some machines with narrow chart paper give

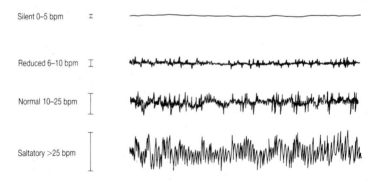

Fig. 11.4. *Baseline variability; band width.*

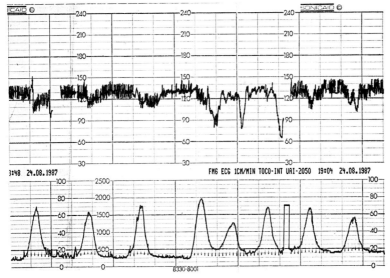

Fig. 11.5. *Artefactual baseline variability.*

a false impression of reduced baseline variability. When reduced variability is recognised, the following factors should be considered:
- Effect of narcotic analgesics
- Effect of sedatives
- Effect of antihypertensives
- Fetal sleep pattern

Fetal sleep patterns are very common, typically occurring as 20–30 minute periods of reduced variability, even late in labour. Reduced variability in the absence of the above causes and in the presence of meconium staining of the amniotic fluid and decelerations is a serious sign of fetal asphyxia.

Artefact of the type shown in Fig. 11.5 should not be mistaken for variability; it may disguise reduced variability and may be corrected by reversing the wires in the leg plate or replacing the electrode. The significance of a saltatory fetal heart pattern showing excessive variability is not clear (Fig. 11.6). It may reflect acute circulatory instability possibly preceding asphyxia.

Accelerations: Accelerations are increases in the fetal heart rate of 15 b.p.m. from the baseline for 15 seconds. Two or more should be present in a 20 minute period to be defined *reactive* and normal (Fig.

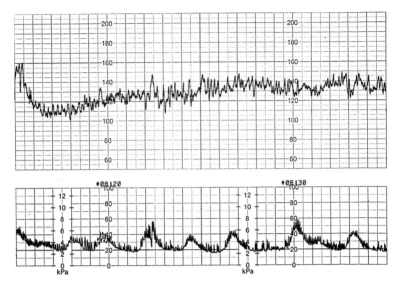

Fig. 11.6. *Saltatory pattern.*

11.7). They do not occur during periods of fetal sleep. Excessive reactivity may lead to confusion with a pattern of baseline tachycardia complicated by decelerations (Fig. 11.8). These can be distinguished by identifying the baseline and inspecting the nature of the peaks and troughs. Excessive reactivity is also associated with many fetal movements usually recorded on the trace.

Baseline reflex activity: (Fig. 11.9) Short, sharp decelerations are often noted on a reactive trace. These reflex signs usually reflect changes in rate precipitated by fetal movement, iatrogenic stimulation and fetal activity. They may be more frequent and pronounced in the preterm fetus.

Decelerations: Early, late, variable or combined.
• Early: onset and recovery coinciding with onset and offset of contractions. They are generally due to head compression if labour progress is normal and amniotic fluid is normal (Fig. 11.10).
• Late: decelerations which commence after the onset of a contraction and finish after it. Usually the onset, trough and recovery are all out of phase. Such decelerations are suggestive of asphyxia, especially when associated with meconium staining of amniotic fluid reduced variability, abnormal rate and show recovery (Fig. 11.11).

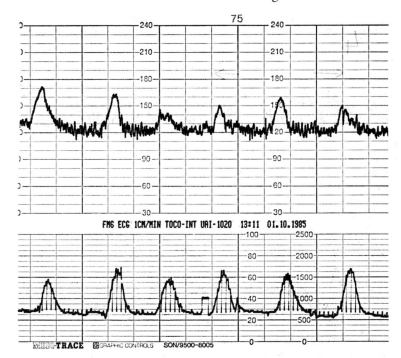

Fig. 11.7. *Reactive trace.*

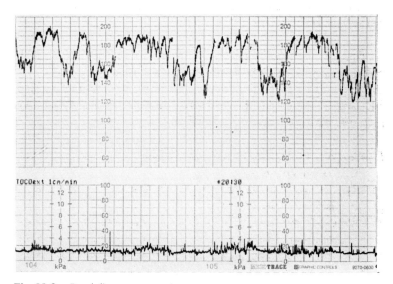

Fig. 11.8. *Pseudodistress; very reactive trace.*

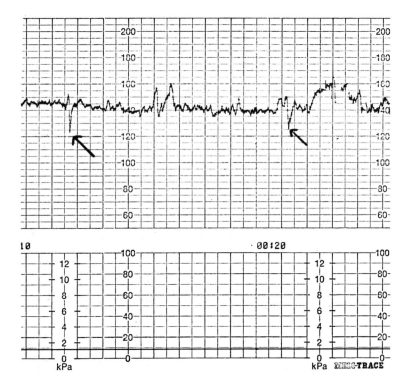

Fig. 11.9. *Baseline reflex activity.*

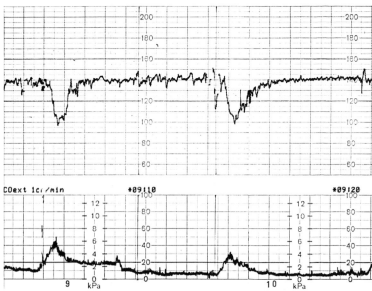

Fig. 11.10. *Early decelerations.*

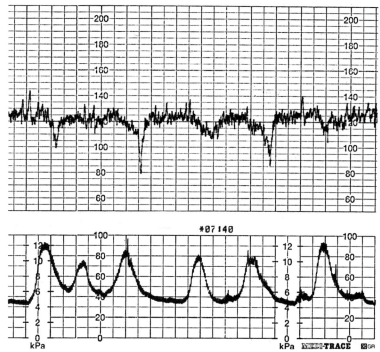

Fig. 11.11. *Late decelerations.*

- Variable: variable decelerations are variable in shape and/or timing. Such decelerations are usually due to cord compression and are relatively benign. However, associated features of variable decelerations must be considered (Fig. 11.12). Persistence of variable decelerations often leads to increasing asphyxial features indicating depleted reserves.

Whilst the above categorisation of traces is descriptive, an analysis of any trace for pathological features is more useful. The essence of a 'benign' deceleration is that it occurs against background features of normal rate and normal variability (Fig. 11.13).

Pathological features of decelerations (Fig. 11.12):
- Late onset
- Slow recovery
- Loss of variability within deceleration
- Absent pre- and post-deceleration acceleration
- Exaggerated post-deceleration acceleration

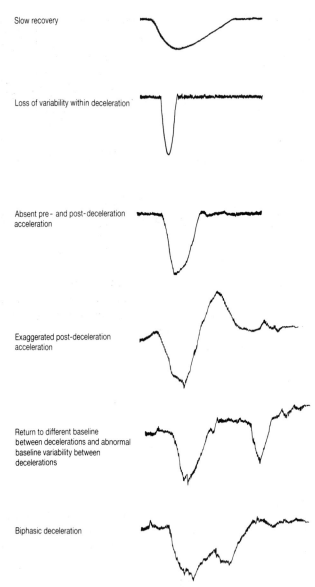

Slow recovery

Loss of variability within deceleration

Absent pre - and post-deceleration acceleration

Exaggerated post-deceleration acceleration

Return to different baseline between decelerations and abnormal baseline variability between decelerations

Biphasic deceleration

Fig. 11.12. *Pathological features of variable decelerations.*

- Return to different baseline after deceleration
- Abnormal baseline variability between decelerations
- Biphasic deceleration

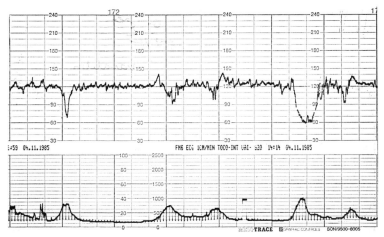

Fig. 11.13. *Variable decelerations without asphyxial features.*

This concept is particularly useful in assessing variable decelerations. The presence of such features suggests impaired autonomic control and asphyxia. Obsession with early or late timing of a deceleratory pattern is simplistic and unreasonable. Appreciation of these more subtle elements is important (see Appendix 1).

Reversible causes of abnormal FHR:
- Dorsal position (supine hypotension)
- Bed pan effect
- Vaginal examination
- Artificial rupture of the membranes
- Epidural insertion or top up
- Oxytocic drugs
- Other drugs especially narcotics

The first step in the management of an abnormal fetal heart rate tracing is to correct the above. If there is any doubt about the nature of the abnormality, the simple expedient of listening with the Pinard stethoscope must *never* be forgotten. If the abnormality persists then further action should be taken:
- Is vaginal delivery imminent and easy? Expedite
- Is vaginal delivery imminent but complicated? Consider checking pH and expedite
- Is vaginal delivery not imminent but prospect of it good? Check fetal pH and review

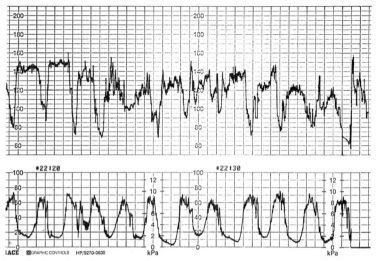

Fig. 11.14. *Second stage normal trace.*

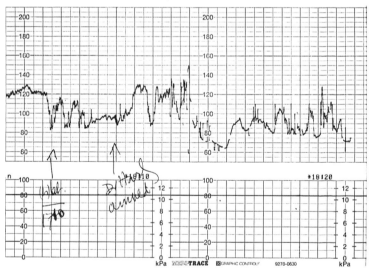

Fig. 11.15. *Second stage abnormal trace.*

• Is vaginal delivery not imminent, prospect poor or other complicating factors present? Consider caesarean section

Fresh, thick meconium staining of the amniotic fluid associated with an abnormal trace is a particularly ominous sign in early labour.

Repeated attempts to obtain a fetal blood sample are inappropriate under these circumstances; delivery is preferable by caesarean section.

The interpretation of second stage traces is modified. Early deceleration of progressive depth are common and benign. The onset of late first stage and second stage may be suspected from the cardiotocograph when these signs appear (Fig. 11.14). If late, or prolonged decelerations appear, or abnormal baseline variability supervenes, then it is potentially significant and delivery should be expedited (Fig. 11.15).

FETAL pH

This is measured in a scalp sample, which is possible when the cervix is dilated enough to accept an amnioscope and the presenting part is relatively fixed. It is performed when there is doubt about the significance of an abnormal fetal heart rate pattern.

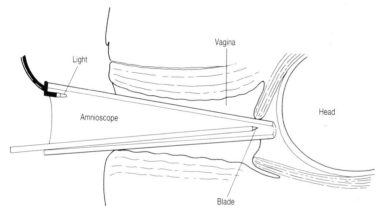

Fig. 11.16. *Fetal blood sampling technique.*

After insertion of the amnioscope (Fig. 11.16), the target area is cleared of mucus, amniotic fluid, or other debris. Ethyl chloride spray is used to dilate the capillary blood vessels. Some vaseline is applied to prevent the blood spreading and a small blade used to stab the scalp. A small amount of blood, free of air bubbles, is drawn up into the capillary tube. This sample is then analysed for pH and, preferably, base excess. Most modern (and expensive) blood gas analysers can give results on small blood samples; about 50 μl in volume.

pH values:
- < 7.20 acidosis: deliver
- 7.20–7.25, repeat after 30 minutes and review
- >7.25, observe trace: repeat if it deteriorates

Too much reliance should not be placed on pH measurement. A normal pH should be interpreted in conjunction with base excess and P_{CO_2}. Research has shown direct measurement of lactate to be the most sensitive biochemical indicator of asphyxia.

CORD BLOOD ANALYSIS

If delivery has been expedited because of an abnormal fetal heart rate tracing or confirmed acidosis, then cord blood analysis for blood gases and pH is desirable. The umbilical cord contains two arteries and one vein. Extraction of a sample from the vein is easy. To obtain a specimen from the artery requires the cord to be double clamped soon after delivery. Failure to do this results in the artery contracting in spasm, and obtaining a sample is difficult. In view of the unreliability of Apgar scores in measuring neonatal outcome and morbidity, routine umbilical cord blood gases should be performed. As umbilical artery blood reflects fetal metabolism better than vein blood, it is preferable, but more difficult, to obtain. Normal values are illustrated below.

Table 11.1 Cord blood gas values.

Normal ranges	Umbilical vein	Umbilical artery
P_{O_2} (mmHg)	24–32	14–22
P_{CO_2} (mmHg)	33–43	43–60
pH	7.26–7.40	7.24–7.35
Base excess (mmol/l)	−2−−17	−2−−17

FETAL 'DISTRESS'

When extensive fetal heart rate monitoring was first introduced, the rate of caesarean deliveries increased, and some babies delivered for 'fetal distress' were born in excellent condition. This implies a high false-positive rate in diagnosing fetal asphyxia by trace analysis. This may be reduced by:

1 Skilled interpretation
2 Fetal pH analysis

There is therefore a difference between an abnormal fetal heart rate tracing, fetal 'distress' and fetal acidosis. Fetal distress is a poor, imprecise term. Simple description of an abnormal fetal heart rate pattern with or without asphyxial features is preferable. Other methods like electrocardiogram wave form analysis, fetal response to stimulation, vibro-acoustic stimulation, electromechanical intervals or blood flow may be important in the future.

See Appendix 1 for further examples of interesting fetal heart rate tracings.

12

Contraction Monitoring

Uterine contractions are crucial in the process of labour and delivery. Efficient powers are essential for progression of labour, but the passenger should not be compromised by them. A well-grown, healthy fetus tolerates this stress, but a hypoxic, small fetus may become further asphyxiated. Hence the importance of fetal heart rate monitoring, especially when oxytocics are used. What information is required about contractions? They should be described as in Fig. 12.1. Traditionally, using information obtained from the palpating hand or external tocographic transducer, their duration, frequency and strength are noted. However, this is not the crux of the matter. What is important is whether the contractions are causing progressive changes in the cervix, especially dilatation. If the fetal heart is normal and the cervix is dilating, no further information is required. Conversely, contractions appearing regularly and frequently on the tocographic tracing may not be painful and may not mean the woman

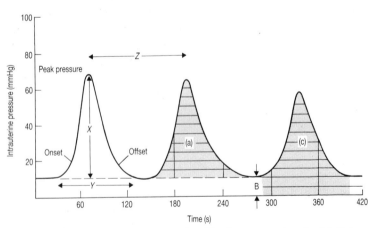

Fig. 12.1. *Terminology of uterine contractions.* X active pressure (amplitude); Y duration; Z contraction interval (related to frequency); (a) active contraction area; B basal tone; (c) total contraction area.

is in labour. This is seen not infrequently on an admission cardiotocograph and must not be misinterpreted as labour, with consequent mistakes in management. For this reason, such patients should not be observed intensively, lying flat in bed but encouraged to ambulate with a 'hands-off' approach adopted by the staff. Ambulation has not been shown to improve labour, but may interrupt a cycle of anxiety.

ABNORMAL CONTRACTIONS

It is in the woman with abnormal labour progress, especially with a poor response to oxytocin, that more detailed assessment of contractions is necessary. External tocography provides only limited information about contraction strength and this is more accurately obtained by measuring uterine pressure with an intrauterine pressure catheter. A disposable, cheap, fluid-filled catheter is slightly difficult to handle and the maintenance of the continuous fluid column can be troublesome. Conversely, the electronic, transducer-tipped catheter (Sonicaid, Gaeltec; Fig. 12.2 & 12.3) is fragile and expensive, but easier to use. There are fewer fetal complications with the latter. Fig. 12.4 shows the methods of contraction monitoring.

How should contractions be measured? Frequency, duration and amplitude may vary independently, making sequential assessment complicated. The concept of the area under the curve has been adopted; the uterine activity integral (UAI) (Fig. 12.5). The area under the curve is computed using the Système International (SI) unit of pressure, the pascal, as the reference. Kilopascal-seconds (kPa.s) per 15 minutes are measured by the Sonicaid FM6 fetal monitor. Fig. 12.6 shows a good quality internal tracing including printed data sequential to a poor quality external tracing. The indications for intrauterine pressure assessment are:

1 Difficult augmentation
2 Difficult stimulation or induction
3 Previous caesarean section with use of oxytocin
4 Breech with use of oxytocin
5 Grand multiparity with use of oxytocin

Should all cases having oxytocin drugs have intrauterine pressure measurement? A case may be made for this, but a proportion of cases respond readily to a low dose of oxytocin (12 milliunits per minute or 4 units per litre at 60 drops per minute) not needing

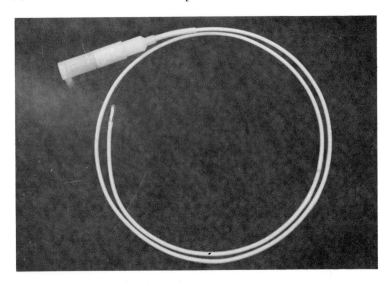

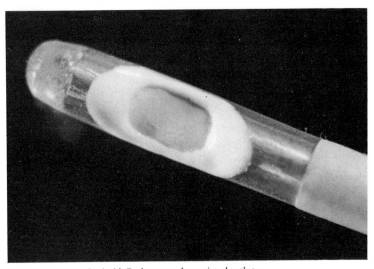

Fig. 12.2–12.3. *Sonicaid-Gaeltec transducer-tipped catheter.*

escalation to higher doses; these cases can be safely managed without measurement of intrauterine pressure. It is the escalation of oxytocin to a higher concentration that implies that an induction or augmentation is difficult.

Different patterns of contractions have different implications for

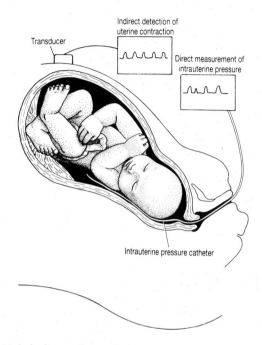

Fig. 12.4. *Methods of contraction monitoring.*

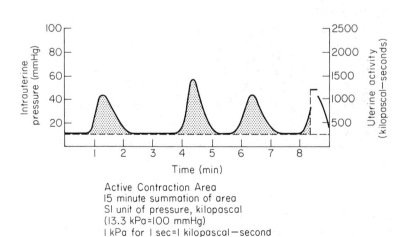

Active Contraction Area
15 minute summation of area
SI unit of pressure, kilopascal
(13.3 kPa=100 mmHg)
1 kPa for 1 sec=1 kilopascal−second
UAI=Active contraction area/15 minutes

Fig. 12.5. *Uterine activity integral (UAI).*

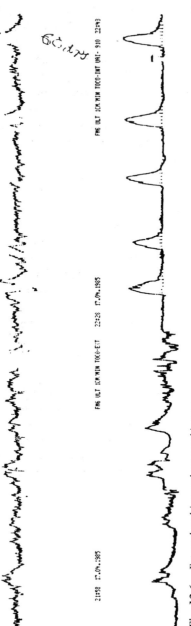

Fig. 12.6. *External and internal tocographic trace.*

labour and the fetus. Hypotonic conventionally means contractions of low amplitude; a contraction amplitude of less than 40 mmHg is unlikely to be associated with normal labour progress. The UAI in these circumstances will be less than 1200 kPa.s $(15 \text{ min})^{-1}$. There is a gradual rise of activity throughout labour and a substantial rise in the late first stage and second stage. The aim should be to generate contractions of between 1500 and 2000 kPa.s $(15 \text{ min})^{-1}$.

Contractions with a frequency greater than 5 per 10 minutes, when oxytocin is being used, represent hyperstimulation (tachysystole) and the oxytocin should be reduced. Hyperstimulation may also manifest as a hypertonic episode; this is seen as a raised basal pressure persisting for several minutes between contractions. It also results from misuse of oxytocin and may be reversed by discontinuing the infusion. Whilst inco-ordination of contractions is seen occasionally in normal progressive labour, it should be considered abnormal when seen in oxytocin-treated labour, often manifesting as coupling or tripling of contractions. Under these circumstances it represents hyperstimulation and the oxytocin should be reduced. The principle of manipulating oxytocin against the endpoint of measured contractions is an obvious one. There is a possible place for the use of beta-mimetic drugs in the management of the patient with excessive uterine activity. Indeed, in centres where anaesthetic support is weak, serious consideration should be given to the use of such drugs in the delay ensuing between decision for caesarean section and the operation itself.

The purpose of internal pressure monitoring is to facilitate the completion of a well conducted labour in a reasonable time, to avoid unnecessary caesarean section because of inadequate oxytocin treatment, and, conversely, avoid iatrogenic fetal asphyxia because of overdosage with oxytocin. Limitation of the time spent in abnormal labour—a time of risk to mother and fetus—is achieved.

13

Second Stage of Labour and Episiotomy

The management of the second stage of labour has become topical in recent years with wider use of epidural analgesia and more frequent vaginal examination.

Although the second stage is recognized to start at full dilatation, the concept of a passive and an active stage is useful. The cervix may be fully dilated, the woman have no urge to push, the presenting part not be seen on parting the labia, and the head be in a transverse position. Pushing is futile under these circumstances and may lead to progressive fetal acidosis. The woman should turn to a lateral position, oxytocin should be given if the contractions are weak, and the initial part of the second stage be conducted passively, without pushing. If an epidural is in place, a full top-up should not be given. If necessary, a 'sitting-up' top-up can be given for perineal pain. When the presenting part becomes visible, the active second stage should begin. Passivity is only appropriate when the fetal heart rate is normal. Second stage augmentation is the key to limiting the forceps delivery rate under these circumstances. As the Dublin School states, 'babies are much better born by propulsion than traction'.

Rigid restriction of the length of the second stage is no longer applied. If the fetal heart rate is normal and some progress is being made, then the second stage should continue. Progress is more difficult to judge in the second stage because it is a matter of descent. However, the presenting part should be visible and be seen to advance perceptibly. It is under these circumstances that examination *during* a contraction is useful.

EPISIOTOMY

Fewer episiotomies have been performed in recent years. It is one area where routine action has been re-examined in the light of changing patient attitudes and criticism of the 'unkindest cut of all'. Several studies have shown that spontaneous tears heal as well as deliberate cuts and there may be less morbidity. Episiotomy remains an integral part of delivery hastened for fetal distress, assisted delivery and preterm delivery. Under normal circumstances, it is only performed when the head is so advanced that the perineum is showing signs of imminent tearing; the woman and attending staff having agreed in advance on its use. If the baby remains undelivered for several contractions after an episiotomy has been cut, then it has been done too early.

Types of episiotomy

The midline episiotomy (Fig. 13.1, label a) has been shown to heal better with less sequelae than its mediolateral counterpart (lable c). However, extension to the anus is a concern and a case can be made for retaining the latter when the baby is large, in an occipito-posterior position or when an assisted delivery is being performed. A J-shaped episiotomy is a compromise (label b).

Episiotomies and tears should be repaired with fine suture material preferably Vicryl, or Dexon. A subcuticular stitch for skin closure is preferable. Simple analgesia is sufficient and there is no evidence that local foams or creams produce a more satisfactory result.

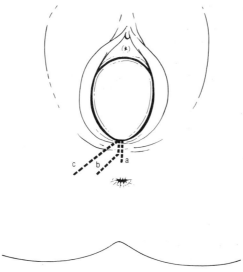

Fig. 13.1. *Types of episiotomy.*

Assisted Delivery and Caesarean Section

The indications for assisted vaginal delivery are:
1 Fetal compromise
2 Maternal distress
3 Failure to progress in the second stage
4 Aftercoming head of a breech
Failure to progress in the second stage may be a manifestation of poor maternal effort, poor contractions, a tight cephalopelvic fit, transverse arrest of the head or persistent occipito-posterior position.

NON-ROTATIONAL

Forceps with a cephalic and a pelvic curve are used for non-rotational delivery as may be the vacuum extractor. In the United Kingdom there is a preference for the former whilst in Scandinavia, the Netherlands and other countries, for the latter. What matters is personal experience and familiarity; both methods are safe in skilled hands.

ROTATIONAL

Kiellands forceps are used in the United Kingdom and the vacuum extractor in other countries for malrotation of the head. Rotational delivery requires particular care and experience. Caution should be exercised when there is an abnormal cardiotocograph as well as a malposition. If rotation is going to be in any way complicated then it is prudent to check the fetal pH first.

PREREQUISITES FOR ASSISTED DELIVERY

- Good contractions
- Membranes ruptured
- Bladder and rectum empty
- Effective analgesia

- Head engaged; 1/5 palpable abdominally at most and below the ischial spines vaginally
- Experienced operator
- Paediatrician present

Babies are much better born by propulsion than extraction. Time should be taken, if necessary, to increase the oxytocin. Some massage of the vagina and perineum seems to stimulate a reflex increase in the expulsive effort and spontaneous delivery may occur.

A major degree of moulding and caput formation is a bad prognostic sign, especially if rotation is required. The obvious implication is that there is a very tight fit and delivery will be difficult and possibly traumatic.

TRIAL OF FORCEPS

If the operator has any doubt about vaginal delivery, then it must be performed in the operating theatre with the anaesthetist and theatre staff present and ready for caesarean section. The episiotomy must not be done until it becomes clear that vaginal delivery will be possible. The worst result is a scar on the perineum as well as on the abdomen with a scarred psyche as a likely concomitant. Failed forceps should be an unusual event if proper assessment has been undertaken.

CAESAREAN SECTION

This is undertaken when there is reason to believe that vaginal delivery entails increased risk to mother or baby. The rate of caesarean section varies from 5% to greater than 20%. Attitudes to the management of breech presentation, fetal distress and pre-term labour affect the rate only slightly. Attitudes to the management of labour and difficult labour (dystocia) are more important. Management of labour with a uterus previously scarred by caesarean section then becomes an added factor in areas with high rates.

Caesarean section may be:

- Elective
- Semi-elective
- Emergency
- Immediate

Elective

This is a planned procedure in cases such as nulliparous breech, repeat caesarean section, etc. It is performed at about 38 weeks' gestation because any greater length of gestation increases the possibility of undesirable spontaneous labour and emergency caesarean section. Performing it sooner increases the risk of neonatal respiratory distress syndrome (RDS) and, particularly, transient tachypnoea of the newborn (TTN). Epidural analgesia is ideal for these cases.

Semi-elective

This case is neither an elective nor an emergency procedure. However, it does have an element of planning. It is usually performed pre-term in conditions such as pre-eclampsia where a steadily deteriorating situation makes it inevitable. Either epidural or general anaesthesia may be appropriate in these cases.

Emergency

Such a procedure may be indicated before labour, but more commonly, during labour due to a complication. A good example is when dystocia is due to cephalo-pelvic disproportion and a trial of labour has failed to bring about delivery. However, the fetal heart is often normal. Undue haste is unnecessary, sometimes dangerous. However, the baby should be delivered in 30–60 minutes. General anaesthesia is usually more appropriate in these cases. An existing epidural may be adjusted.

Immediate

This is urgent. It is performed for acute fetal compromise, placental abruption, or cord prolapse. The person taking the decision, usually during vaginal examination, inserts a urinary catheter. The anaesthetist is summoned, pubic shaving dispensed with, and urgent, immediate delivery performed. It should be possible for the decision to delivery interval to be less than 12 minutes. If it is more, then procedures should be re-examined.

The fetal heart should be auscultated shortly before any caesarean section. If necessary, for instance in concealed abruption, a real time ultrasound scan just before starting the operation is useful.

Incisions

The skin incision for caesarean section is transverse suprapubic (label a), midline subumbilical (label b) or rarely, paramedian above and below the umbilicus (label c) (Fig. 14.1). Classical caesarean section is now uncommon. However, a woman coming from a developing country with a paramedian scar may have had one. The skin incision is not otherwise indicative of the type of caesarean section. A transverse suprapubic incision is now most common in the United Kingdom with better results. The uterine incision (Fig. 14.2, label a) is usually transverse lower segment. True classical (label c) is now very rare. However, a lower midline uterine incision (label b) has a place in the delivery of the very pre-term baby, especially by the breech, with oliogohydramnios and transverse lie. When a greater deal of investment has been made in a high-risk pregnancy, it is disastrous

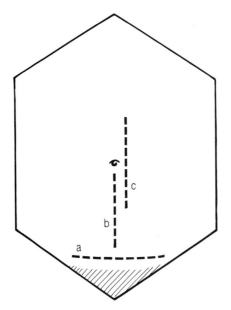

Fig. 14.1. *Skin incisions for caesarean section.*

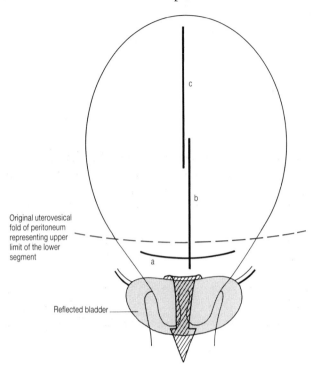

Original uterovesical
fold of peritoneum
representing upper
limit of the lower
segment

Reflected bladder

Fig. 14.2.   *Uterine incisions at caesarean section.*

to damage the very small baby during delivery itself through a poorly
formed tight lower segment. The decision to use such a uterine
incision is *only* made after the peritoneal cavity has been opened and
the uterine shape assessed. There are obvious implications for a future
pregnancy when some would regard it as a classical scar. This area
requires further study.

15
Ultrasound

Mobile, real time ultrasound equipment has only been available since 1980. As with any new technology its role should be identified or it will be misused. Two basic principles apply.

1 It should *not* be used when the same or better result is obtained by clinical or other means.

2 It should be used only when a trained operator is capable of obtaining the desired result recognised to be within the limits of the machine.

The machine currently available which lends itself most readily to use in the labour ward is the Pye Medical Scanner 400 (Fig. 15.1). Emergency ultrasound has a role to play in the following clinical situations:

- Intrauterine fetal death (IUD)
- Uncertain presentations:
  obesity
  pre-term
- Multiple pregnancy:
  diagnosis
  fetal size
  presentation
- Pre-term labour:
  size
  presentation
  normality
  fetal breathing
- Rupture of membranes (pre-term):
  amniotic fluid volume
  amniocentesis
- Vaginal bleeding:
  placental localization

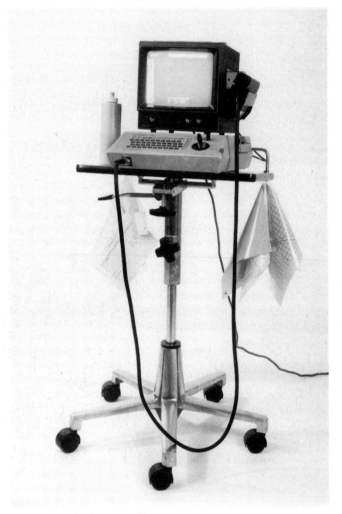

Fig. 15.1. *Pye Medical Scanner 400.*

INTRAUTERINE DEATH (IUD)

This diagnosis is not a true obstetric emergency, except in acute asphyxial conditions. However, the ability to reassure a couple about the presence of a fetal heart when the ultrasound department is closed is desirable. Under acute circumstances it may be crucial. Clinical

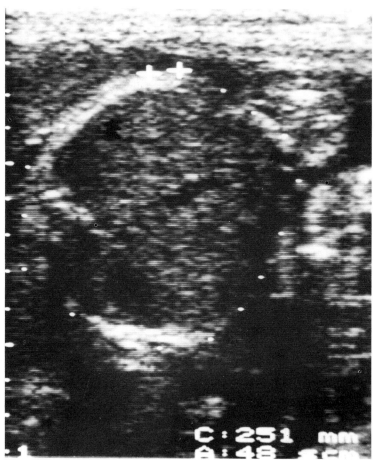

Fig. 15.2. *Abdominal circumference (AC) on ultrasound.*

auscultation and recording with an electronic monitor is impossible when the uterus is tense and tender with a concealed abruption. Evidence of a fetal heart beat is important prior to caesarean section. Traditional palpation of the prolapsed cord is also unreliable and visualized action of the central pump may be crucial. Potential survivors may be born with an Apgar score of zero but only if the fetal heart disappeared in the immediately preceding period and other adverse factors are not present.

PRESENTATION

In the obese patient or pre-term labour accurate assessment of presentation and multiple pregnancy is impossible without a scan. In active labour this is important.

The place of emergency ultrasound will reflect to some extent the existing ultrasound services. If one scan is standard in every pregnancy then in all booked cases dating, exclusion of multiple pregnancy, exclusion of major abnormality and placental localization will already have been done.

PRE-TERM LABOUR

A woman presenting with threatened pre-term labour between 24 and 32 weeks will be difficult to assess clinically. Ultrasound permits determination of presentation, size, normality and the presence or absence of fetal breathing. Measurement of the fetal abdominal circumference (Fig. 15.2) and biparietal diameter are plotted on a weight estimate chart (Appendix 2). The association of abnormality and pre-term labour has been proposed, and reassurance about normality, especially prior to caesarean section, is important. The dilemma over the use of tocolytics remains, and significant placebo response is common. There is evidence that in the absence of multiple pregnancy, rupture of the membranes, and bleeding, the presence of fetal breathing means pre-term delivery will not occur within 48 hours. This could be used to justify withholding tocolysis. Ultrasound guided amniocentesis is useful when there is a history suggestive of membrane rupture and the scan appearance is suggestive of reduced amniotic fluid volume.

ANTEPARTUM HAEMORRHAGE

In cases not previously scanned, the ability to exclude placenta praevia may be important under emergency circumstances. On the contrary, ultrasound should not be used to look for retroplacental clot in the same context; there is an appreciable rate of false-negative findings. A major abruption requiring delivery is usually clinically obvious and scanning only delays delivery. Control must be exercised on the use and role of ultrasound in the labour ward.

16

Neonatal Management

ANNE GREENOUGH

Transition from fetal to independent neonatal life is perhaps the most important and difficult adaptation any of us make. As a consequence it is not surprising that those first important hours after birth can include serious, often life-threatening problems. Most immediate is the delivery of an asphyxiated infant that requires appropriate and speedy resuscitation. Second is the recognition of congenital abnormalities, or possibility injuries, related to the birth process which require immediate attention. To ensure that this important period goes smoothly requires detailed knowledge of the physiological processes which occur in the adaptive process, skills of resuscitation and the ability to distinguish abnormal from normal in the newborn.

Ideally, all infants should be delivered in a situation where they have immediate access to personnel skilled in resuscitation and care of the newborn. Certainly, those infants in whom compromise has already been predicted or demonstrated should be given the benefit of a skilled 'resuscitator' attending the delivery. The appropriate equipment must be available.

A liaison ward round between obstetricians and paediatricians involved in these high-risk pregnancies should be carried out so that the neonatal intensive care unit is always up to date with high-risk mothers.

PHYSIOLOGICAL CHANGES AT BIRTH

The first breath results from various stimuli: hypoxia, acidosis, temperature change and occlusion of the umbilical cord. The first few breaths see the formation of functional residual capacity and, over the subsequent hours, reabsorption of lung liquid occurs. The pulmonary vascular resistance decreases as a response to the first breath and lung expansion causes closure of the foramen ovale due to pressure changes within the heart and constriction of the ductus arteriosus in response to increased oxygenation. These changes, plus the loss of placental circulation, result in transition from the fetal to the adult type circulation. They can, however, be reversed in response to asphyxia during the first days of life.

SEQUENCE OF RESPONSES TO ASPHYXIA

- Increased respiratory effort—heart rate and blood pressure maintained
- Primary apnoea—heart rate >100
- Pain, cold, analeptics, tactile and thermal stimuli will all initiate respiration in primary apnoea*
- Gasping
- Last gasp, heart rate and blood pressure fall
- Terminal (secondary) apnoea—heart rate <100

In secondary apnoea, above stimuli (*) are useless, only positive pressure inflation is successful in resuscitation.

Timing of this sequence of responses can be modified; for example, narcotics decrease respiratory efforts and therefore prolong primary apnoea, whereas hypothermia prolongs the period of gasping. It should always be remembered that asphyxial insults may, and can, have occurred prior to delivery, therefore the infant may be delivered in terminal apnoea requiring immediate intubation for resuscitation.

ASSESSMENT OF ASPHYXIA

Table 16.1   Apgar score.

Clinical features	Score		
	0	1	2
Heart rate	Absent	<100	>100
Respiration	Absent	Gasping or irregular	Regular
Muscle tone	Limp	Diminished	Normal
Response of pharyngeal catheter	Nil	Grimace	Cough
Colour of trunk	White	Blue	Pink

Apgar score is traditionally calculated at 1, 5 and 10 minutes and, by scoring cardiorespiratory status, can give a guide to the degree of asphyxia and resuscitation need;

- 7–10 indicates a vigorous infant, no resuscitation required.
- 4–6 a mild to moderately depressed infant—some form of resuscitation is required (infant pale blue with a heart rate <100, inadequate respiration).
- 0–3 pale, cyanotic, apnoeic, hyptonic infant with reduced or absent reflex response—immediate positive pressure ventilation is essential.

CAUSES OF ASPHYXIA

Maternal

- Compression of the inferior vena cava or aorta by the gravid uterus
- Uterine hypertonus
- Low blood pressure—blood loss, pharmacological agents, lack of ventilation
- Anaemia
- Abnormal placental function (too small, separation, infarcts)

Fetal

- Mechanical occlusion of the umbilical cord
- Depressant drugs

Neonatal

- Depressant drugs
- Immaturity
- Meconium aspiration
- Congenital abnormalities

Indication for paediatrician at delivery (or medical personnel skilled at resuscitation of infant who is only responsible for his/her care):
- Anaesthesia/analgesia, e.g. caesarean section
- Instrumental delivery, e.g. forceps
- Multiple birth
- Breech

- Prematurity
- Antepartum haemorrhage (APH)
- Signs of fetal compromise:
  cardiotocograph abnormalities
  meconium stained liquor
- Abnormality of the infant anticipated, e.g. rhesus disease, prematurity
- Other obstetric complications

It is vital to have adequate warning if such a delivery is anticipated. Immediately prior to the delivery, resuscitation equipment should be checked by the person responsible for the care of the infant. In addition resuscitation equipment should be checked daily by labour ward personnel. The paediatrician attending the delivery should run through the following sequence:

- Check oxygen supply, blow off valve (30 cm H_2O) functioning, bag and mask (series of masks appropriate to size of baby).
- Facilities for intubation, e.g. selection of endotracheal tubes, nasal and oral as to preference and expertise.
- Check; all connectors fit, laryngoscope with working bulb, McGill's forceps if nasal intubation is contemplated, working suction.
- Temperature control—overhead heater functioning. Avoidance of hypothermia is essential—this decreases surfactant function, worsening respiratory distress.
- Equipment for difficult resuscitation, e.g. facilities for umbilical cannulation. Equipment present for both thoracocentesis and paracentesis.
- Drugs; saline, both for irrigation of endotracheal tube in meconium aspiration (see below), and for flushing of umbilical catheter. Bicarbonate, adrenaline, dextrose, calcium gluconate, atropine.

CRITERIA FOR INTUBATION

- Heart rate <100 (indicative of secondary or terminal apnoea); immediate intubation and positive pressure inflation.
- Inadequate or no respiratory efforts after two minutes despite maintenance of heart rate.
- Prematurity? <28 weeks gestation (unless vigorous respiratory effort) intubate and achieve cardiorespiratory stability and transfer

intubated (and ventilated if necessary) to the neonatal intensive care unit. There, with good monitoring, the decision can be made to extubate.

ACTIVE RESUSCITATION

In secondary apnoea, positive pressure inflation is necessary to re-establish spontaneous respiration. This can be achieved either by bag and mask or via endotracheal tube. Using a bag and mask, prolonged inflation cannot be achieved, therefore endotracheal intubation and positive pressure inflation provide the most effective and safe method of resuscitation.

AT DELIVERY

The action necessary is dependent on the infant's condition at birth (see below).

Fit, healthy baby, crying, pink, heart rate >100

No resuscitation necessary. Vitamin K administered according to policy. Unncessary suction of the nose or pharynx can increase vagal stimulation and result in bradycardia and apnoea. Maintain temperature as a cold infant may develop signs of respiratory distress (grunting) as a result of reduced surfactant function.

Heart rate >100 but respiration inadequate

- Transfer baby to resuscitaire. Dry and keep warm.
- Oxygen via a face mask and assess patency of airway—good response, no further action.
- Analgesia prior to delivery—naloxone—good response, continue to observe as the half life of naloxone is short.
- Heart rate falls despite oxygen—intubation and positive pressure inflation till regular heart rate and respiration is established—extubate and observe. (i) Poor or irregular respiration—reintubate and transfer to special care baby unit (SCBU) intubated (ventilated if necessary). (ii) Respiration maintained following extubation with a good heart rate. After observation for about 1 hour, transfer to ward with mother.

Heart rate <100 no respiratory effort

Clear airway, intubate immediately.

Procedure for intubation; minimal hyperextension is necessary. Insert laryngoscope into right hand corner of mouth, pushing the tongue towards the left between the blade and the left hand corner of the mouth. Avoid excessive force on the upper gum. Pass the blade between the tongue and the epiglottis and elevate the tip to reveal the glottis. The tube should be advanced approximately 2 cm below the cords (nasotracheal tube clearly marked). Inflation pressures; term infant 30 cm H_2O, pre-term infant 18–20 cm H_2O. After the first few inflations it may be possible to turn down the peak pressure; assess by watching chest wall excursion. Ensure position of endo-tracheal tube, listen for bilateral symmetrical noises and watch for expansion of chest. Expansion of stomach or louder sounds in the abdomen of air entry indicates oesophageal intubation. Asymetrical breath sounds—endotracheal tube in the right main bronchus; pneumothorax.

Good response to intubation, heart rate >100, pink; regular respiration commences—extubation and period of observation on the labour ward.

Good heart rate and pink, but no respiratory effort isusually due to acidosis—bicarbonate given (see below). Cord pH to be measured in all deliveries where problems are anticipated to occur and in this way an accurate assessment of the degree of acidosis can be obtained. Good response to bicarbonate with regular respiration; extubation and a period of observation but in SCBU.

No or very low fetal heart rate

No respiratory effort. Beware! These infants may be very acidotic and certainly require more than one pair of hands at resuscitation.

Artificial ventilation commenced immediately.

Cardiac massage middle and lower third of the sternum using index and middle finger or place both hands encircling the chest so that sternum is compressed by both thumbs. Ratio of massage : inflation=4 : 1.

Catheterization of the umbilical vein (repeated drug administration by direct injection not recommended as multiple puncture sites may lead to bleeding, spasm and failure of drugs to reach the circulation).
• Give alkali 2 ml per kg. $NaHCO_3$ and tromethamine (THAM) (both are suitable bases) are hyperosmolar solutions and in pre-term infants associated with intraventricular haemorrhage. They should both, therefore, be diluted and given slowly at 2–3 ml per minute.
• THAM is advantageous if there is respiratory acidosis, e.g. severe respiratory distress syndrome (RDS), but can enter cells and depress respiration. Twice the quantity of THAM is required compared to $NaHCO_3$.
• An ECG lead should be positioned.
• The following sequence of drugs is given:
  i.v. dextrose
  adrenaline 0.5 ml of 1 in 1000
  1 ml calcium gluconate
(cardiac massage and positive pressure inflation continuing).
  If no response repeat sequence but with intracardiac adrenaline. If after 20 minutes no heart rate is seen, resuscitation attempts should be abandoned as neurological prognosis is extremely poor. Heart rate <100, no respiratory efforts at 30 minutes (and no history of pharmacological respiratory depressant) again discontinue resuscitation attempts.
N.B. The decision to stop is difficult and should be taken by a senior member of staff. If necessary, transfer to NICU where the infant can be more accurately assessed. This should also be the policy for an infant suspected of severe congenital abnormality or of being very immature.

PROBLEMS WITH RESUSCITATION

1 *Failure of equipment*, e.g. running out of oxygen.
2 *Failure of intubation* and positive pressure inflation. Insufficient pressure applied, e.g. in severe RDS, Potter's syndrome, pulmonary hypoplasia—assess by watching chest wall excursion. Size of tube may be insufficient; 3 or 3.5 tube should always be used in a term infant. Endotracheal tube incorrectly sited.

3 *Infant may be severely anaemic*, e.g. following APH, hydropic infant (rhesus disease).

4 *Infant may have abnormalities of the lung*

● pneumothorax diagnosed by needle aspiration or cold light source, if available; only after other failures of resuscitation have been excluded.

● diaphragmatic hernia ⎫ diagnosed by chest X-ray.
● pulmonary hypoplasia ⎭

5 *Infant may be severely infected*—remains pale and hypotensive; immediate and urgent exchange transfusion, with blood pressure support and adequate antibiotic cover.

N.B. It is important in such cases to isolate the aetiological organism. Therefore, antibiotics should be withheld from a pyrexial, or suspected infected mother in labour, unless essential as they may interfere with bacterial isolation from the infant.

COMPLICATIONS OF ASPHYXIA

Infants who have been resuscitated following severe asphyxia should be admitted to SCBU. Such infants may develop a number of problems.

● *Neurological*
fits
cerebral oedema
cerebral haemorrhage
● *Cardiovascular*
abnormalities of rhythm
heart failure
fluid overload
hypotension
● *Metabolic*
low calcium
low glucose
inappropriate antidiuretic hormone (ADH)
● *Renal failure*
acute tubular necrosis
● *Respiratory problems*
pulmonary haemorrhage
RDS
● *Clotting problems*

It is important to be aware and to treat these problems immediately, as the majority of even severely asphyxiated infants may recover with the absence of neurological sequelae. Persisting neurological signs later than 4–5 days from birth are a bad prognostic sign.

SPECIAL PROBLEMS

Hydropic infants

Compounding problems:
- anaemia (rhesus disease)
- prematurity
- ascites ⎫ preventing lung expansion.
- pleural effusion ⎭

Immediate intubation.
Remove ascitic fluid (19 or 21-gauge needle into flank).
Anaemia:
- check packed cell volume (PCV)
- transfuse 20 ml per kg
- if heart failure—immediate exchange transfusion may be preferred.

Meconium aspiration

Any delivery with meconium-stained liquor should have a paediatrician in attendance at delivery. Immediately, prior to delivery of trunk, suck out pharynx. After delivery of body place infant on resuscitaire; inspection of airway via direct laryngoscopy.

- Meconium at or below cords; intubate and suction (suction to endotracheal tube may be necessary if meconium is thick, or irrigation with normal saline 0.5–1 ml). Clearing the meconium from airway is more important than the maintenance of the heart rate initially as it is vital to prevent meconium aspiration syndrome.
- No meconium at or near cords; clear nose and mouth if necessary.
- Always suck out stomach, aspiration from the gastric contents may occur later, on the ward

Clamping the chest to prevent respiratory efforts immediately after delivery may be helpful—but is difficult in a very vigorous infant—also chest wall recoil has occurred with the delivery of the chest.

N.B. The important manoeuvre is suction prior to the first breath, then continued and efficient removal of meconium to prevent meconium aspiration syndrome.

Features of *meconium aspiration syndrome*:
- Chemical pneumonitis
- Mechanical obstruction within airways
- *Escherischia coli* infection

NEONATAL ASSESSMENT ON THE LABOUR WARD

There are several purposes of thorough neonatal assessment on the labour ward:

1 To assess the infant is well and ready for transfer to the postnatal ward.

2 The detection of obvious congenital abnormalities or birth injuries that should be pointed out and explained to the mother and appropriate treatment instituted.

3 To pick up early problems requiring further investigation, observation and/or referral to paediatrician (with admittance to SCBU).

The following is a quick check list:

Unusual facies
- Down's syndrome[+]
- Cleft lip[+]

Colour—cyanosis
- Central congenital heart disease[+]
- Differential cyanosis persistent ductus arteriosus (PDA) (shunting involved)[+]
- Peripheral cyanosis indicative of hypothermia; check temperature. N.B. may be confused with bruising

Colour—Pale
- Anaemia (haemoglobin, PCV)[+]
- Asphyxia[+]

Colour—bruising (if extensive, beware later development of jaundice)
- Birth trauma

- Petechiae—viral infection, idiopathic thrombocytopenic purpura (ITP)[‡]

Respiration
- Tachypnoea[‡]
- Respiratory distress (chest X-ray, etc.)[‡]
- Apnoeic episodes[‡]
- Neurological abnormalities[‡]
- Drugs[‡]
- Stridor? post-intubation[‡]

Cardiovascular system
- Presence of peripheral pulses
- Coarctation (b.p. in all four limbs)[‡]
- Heart rate, irregular, supraventricular tachycardia (SVT)–ECG[‡]
- Heart sounds—presence of a murmur; ECG, chest X-ray[‡]

Abdomen
- Ascites, hydrops[‡]
- Umbilical hernia[*]
- Inguinal hernia noted for referral to surgeon[†]
- Concavity of abdomen—suspect diaphragmatic hernia, supine X-ray[‡]
- Kidneys very easy to feel at this stage—enlarged[‡]
- Cord—presence of one umbilical artery associated with renal abnormalities
- Genitalia—possible ambiguity (beware pre-term infants)[‡]
- Descent of testes—not palpable[†]
- Anus—imperforate, appropriate X-ray[‡]

Neurology
- Tone, movement, cry, behaviour, e.g. irritability[‡]

Structural
- Spine—spina bifida, cleft palate[‡]
- Hips—detection of congenital dislocated hips[†]
- Talipes—positional, i.e. correctable to normal[†]
- Head circumference ⎫
- Weight ⎬ plotted on centile charts
- Microcephaly[‡]—(large, plethoric infant, diabetic mother), small

for dates baby (>10th centile); emphasize regular checking by Dextrostix for early detection of hypoglycaemia

Birth injuries
- Bruising, forceps marks.
- *Caput secundum* (not bounded by suture lines, disappears within a few days)[*]
- Cephalhaematoma (bounded by suture lines may take weeks to resolve. Do not needle as this increases the risk of infection).[*]
- Skull fractures—suspect if prolonged delivery, long labour, or forceps delivery. Unusual.[‡]
- Linear fractures; no specific therapy.
- Depressed fractures obvious on clinical examination; immediate neurosurgical consultation.[‡]
- Intracranial haemorrhage. May be totally asymptomatic; alteration of behaviour, irritability, seizures.[‡]
- Facial palsy—prolonged pressure during delivery, forceps delivery, or congenital abnormality[†], e.g. central paralysis (agenesis of the facial nerve nucleus) limited to the lower half, or two thirds of the contralateral side of the face; peripheral paralysis (complete involves the entire side of the face) open eye at rest, mouth is drawn to the normal side on crying. Treatment; protect the eye.
- Fractures of facial bones. Association with forceps delivery, breech presentation. Alleviate respiratory distress. Referral early, as early union occurs following facial fractures. If fracture is reduced and fixed, rapid healing without complication is the usual course.
- Conjunctival haemorrhage—bright red patches on the conjunctiva after difficult delivery; reassurance.[*]
- Fracture of the clavicle—delivery of extended arms, breech delivery.[†] Decreased or absent movement of the arm and the affected side, later deformity and discoloration may be visible. Moro reflex on the affected side is absent. Treatment; minimizing pain, immobilization, if necessary.
- Brachial palsy—mechanical trauma C5–T1 (large infant and dystocia[‡] or breech extraction and excessive traction). Three types:

  1 Erb's; upper arm C5–6; most common. Grasp reflex intact, absent Moro reflex. Abducted, internally rotated, arm flexed at the wrist.

  2 Klumpke's C8–T1; least common. Intrinsic muscles of hand affected plus homolateral.

3 Horner's; entire arm. Fractures of long bone; displacement, mobility, pain.

- Fractures of humerus.[‡]
- Fractures of femur.[‡]

---

[*] Noted, pointed out to parents, and reassurance given.
[†] Noted, checked later and appropriate referral made if necessary.
[‡] For immediate referral to paediatrician and further investigation.

Part 2
Common Emergencies

17

Shoulder Dystocia

This is an important, common obstetric emergency requiring prompt, efficient treatment which may be life-saving. There has been uncertainty about its definition, but if there is difficulty delivering the shoulders with the contraction subsequent to that which delivered the head, this is shoulder dystocia. The following risk factors suggest the possibility of shoulder dystocia.

- Previous shoulder dystocia
- Previous baby >4 kg
- Estimated fetal weight >4 kg
- Dysfunctional labour, prolonged second stage and assisted delivery

Wait for the contraction and, if the shoulders are not delivered, adopt this drill:

- Don't panic; call for help.
- Turn patient on side/lithotomy position.
- Fully flex hips and knees.
- Do/extend episiotomy.
- Try upward pressure and rotation (disimpaction).
- Assistant exerts gentle pressure suprapubically. Operator passes hand to posterior axilla and attempts rotation through 180° pushing spine anteriorly and exerting gentle traction.
- If this fails, then hand is passed along the ventral surface of the fetus until the posterior hand can be grasped. Hand and forearm are then withdrawn over chest past the face. Must be pulled anteriorly.
- Deliberate cleidotomy should not be necessary.
- Do not use fundal pressure.

Gentleness, but firmness is required. If the patient is agitated, in pain and unable to co-operate, a bolus of pethidine 75 mg or diamorphine 5 mg i.v. will help the situation. This is not drastic, but entirely appropriate in these difficult circumstances.

18

Antepartum Haemorrhage

This is defined as any bleeding from the genital tract between the stage of viability and the birth of the baby. Bleeding before the stage of viability is threatened miscarriage, but has a similar underlying pathogenesis. Antepartum haemorrhage (APH) effectively includes intrapartum haemorrhage; bleeding during labour. A show is release of the blood-stained mucus plug. It can occur only once; anything more is a haemorrhage.

The pathogenesis of APH may be:
- Placenta praevia
- Placental abruption
- Local causes
- Indeterminate
- Vasa praevia

The blood lost is always maternal, except in vasa praevia. It is consequently most serious for the fetus in vasa praevia because of the much smaller circulating blood volume of the fetus. Clues to the pathogenesis may be obtained from clinical assessment.

HISTORY

Bleeding from placenta praevia is typically painless, whilst that from significant, concealed abruption is painful. Bleeding from a small abruption, local causes and vasa praevia is painless. Any pathology, but especially a local cervical lesion, is associated with a post-coital timing. Other kinds of trauma, particularly abdominal, may be followed by placental abruption. Bleeding from any cause may be followed by painful contractions, indicating uterine irritability.

EXAMINATION

A soft uterus with a high presenting part or malpresentation strongly suggests placenta praevia. A hard, woody uterus indicates a major degree of abruption. Any significant tenderness also suggests abruption. *Digital examination must not be performed until placenta praevia has been excluded.* A gentle speculum examination may reveal a local lesion or more directly from where the blood is coming. If labour has supervened and the clinical signs do not suggest placenta praevia, then an experienced person should examine digitally and proceed to artificial rupture of the membranes.

MANAGEMENT

Many patients have a small haemorrhage, often before admission. Their management is at the discretion of the clinician. What follows is an account relating to significant major haemorrhage.

HYPOVOLAEMIC SHOCK APH

Tachycardia, hypotension, cold, clammy peripheries and agitation are the signs of this. In the case of concealed placental abruption, the external loss is inconsistent with the degree of shock and there is a quantity of blood in the uterus. *Coagulopathy is likely.* Whatever the underlying pathology, delivery with aggressive resuscitation is in the maternal interest, irrespective of fetal condition. A scan to look for placenta praevia loses valuable time.

- Blood for Hb, group and match, clotting.
- Site intravenous cannula (largest bore).
- Haemaccel, Gelofusin or Hartmann's Solution i.v. quickly, followed by blood.
- Analgesia, if necessary.
- Examine in operating theatre:
  Caesarean section if not in progressive labour and bleeding uncontrolled, circulation unstable.
  Vaginal delivery if presenting part advancing and circulation stable.
  Central venous pressure monitoring and rapid transfusion through a second cannula should be organized concomitantly.

FLUID MANAGEMENT

Control of volume and input of intravenous fluid is crucial, as is recording of urine output through a urinary catheter. Undertransfusion is much commoner and more serious than overtransfusion. Fresh blood is now rarely available, however, packed cells, fresh frozen plasma (FFP), and platelets play a similar role. The use of FFP should be guided by clotting studies. Fibrinogen may occasionally be needed. A major degree of obstetric haemorrhage requires at least 6 units of blood. At this stage platelets are also necessary.

A urine output of 0.5 ml per kg per hour is acceptable. When an adult becomes oliguric, 25 ml or less of urine will be produced hourly. In obstetric haemorrhage, pre-renal hypovolaemia is likely and this may be suspected from a low central venous pressure. Replenishing the circulating volume is necessary before urine output will improve or diuretics have any effect. Various investigations help to elucidate the underlying cause of oliguria:

- Urine specific gravity >1016 suggests pre-renal cause.
- Urine Na^+ >30 mmol per litre suggests intrinsic renal failure.
- Urine urea <185 mmol per litre suggests intrinsic renal failure.
- Urine : plasma-urea ratio, >2 : 1 suggests pre-renal cause.
- Urine : plasma osmolality, >2 : 1 suggests pre-renal cause.

Further discussion is beyond the scope of this book.

INTERMEDIATE DEGREES OF HAEMORRHAGE

In other cases, the patient does not become shocked and the episode of bleeding settles. Aggressive management with central venous cannulation and transfusion is unnecessary. Ultrasound scan is done to guide management. A *major* degree of placenta praevia is functionally one where the edge of the placenta is below the presenting part. Any bleeding from the pregnant uterus *must* be coming from the area of the placenta, whether or not there is placenta praevia. When this occurs at term, delivery should be considered.

VASA PRAEVIA

This is uncommon, but life-threatening to the fetus. An astute observer notices that a small amount of blood loss is associated with a very abnormal fetal heart rate tracing. This may follow rupture of the membranes or vaginal examination. Immediate delivery is indicated without awaiting confirmation that the blood is fetal blood. This, however, should be done as it will help the paediatrician. A very pale baby may be suffering from shock or severe anaemia. In the latter case an immediate blood injection may save its life.

19

Postpartum Haemorrhage and Retained Placenta

Postpartum haemorrhage (PPH) is excessive blood loss after delivery of the baby leading or likely to lead to a rising pulse rate, falling blood pressure and poor peripheral perfusion. Meaningful measurement of blood loss is impossible. PPH remains an important cause of maternal death in the United Kingdom. Rapid effective treatment is crucial and a plan of action is important.

PPH is due to:

- Poor uterine contraction—hypotonic.
- Trauma to the genital tract.
- Coagulopathy, usually secondary to the above or secondary to placental abruption.

Antepartum haemorrhage (APH) is associated with PPH. Table 19.1 shows the associations of different types of haemorrhage.

Table 19.1 Associations of different types of haemorrhage.

Hypotonic	Traumatic	Coagulopathy
Nulliparity	Multiparity	Heavy bleeding
Uterine overdistension multiple pregnancy polyhydramnios large baby fibroids	Assisted delivery forceps vacuum extraction Previous uterine scar	Placental abruption Pre-eclampsia/eclampsia Pre-existing coagulation disorder
Prolonged labour induction augmentation stimulation	Intrauterine manipulation internal version	
Placenta praevia	Vaginal and perineal damage	
Grand multiparity		

MANAGEMENT

- Palpate the uterus abdominally and rub up a contraction.
- Call for help.
- Give ergometrine, 0.5 mg i.v.
- Site intravenous cannula for immediate fluid replacement (see below) and further oxytocics.
- Give 100 units of oxytocin in 1 litre of normal saline at 30 drops per minute (150 milliunits per minute).
- Check perineum and vagina.

If significant further bleeding continues, more detailed examination of the genital tract is necessary, especially if factors associated with trauma listed on preceding page are operative:

- Further 0.5 mg ergometrine i.v.
- Continuous fundal massage.
- Good light, lithotomy and analgesia for detailed vaginal and cervical inspection.
- Repair of trauma as indicated.

If bleeding continues obviously from the uterine cavity:

- Arrange examination under anaesthesia in theatre.
- Check uterine cavity.
- Continue massage bimanually.
- Give intramyometrial oxytocic:
  oxytocin, 5 units
  ergometrine, 0.5 mg
  prostaglandin E_2, 2 mg.
- Give prostaglandin infusion; 5 mg PGE_2 (Prostin) in 500 ml of normal saline at 10 µg per min. (20 drops per minute). Increase as necessary, but contraction should occur.

Continued bleeding requires laparotomy:

- Internal iliac ligation
- Hysterectomy

Uterine packing may be used as a temporary expedient. Any oxytocic drug may be injected directly into the uterus with effect.

Such a plan should only be used in a patient requiring it. Remember, intravenous ergometrine is very unpleasant for the patient. Conversely, the plan must be set in motion early in a patient requiring it. The previously hypertensive patient suffering a PPH has no contraindication to ergometrine.

FLUID REPLACEMENT

Initial infusion may be of Hartmann's solution or normal saline, but a colloid becomes necessary in order to maintain volume within the intravascular space. Haemaccel (Hoechst) or Gelofusine (Consolidated Chemicals), which are both chemically modified solutions of degraded gelatin, is the best choice initially, but should be followed by whole blood and fresh frozen plasma. The only difference between them is that Haemaccel contains over 10 times more calcium than Gelofusine. The calcium can lead to clotting in warming coils when Haemaccel is mixed with citrated blood or fresh frozen plasma. The other options are dextrans which unfortunately lead to problems in blood cross-matching, and Hespan (Du Pont) which is hetastarch and is expensive. In cases of massive, rapid haemorrhage, uncross-matched group O negative blood should be given. In the face of massive haemorrhage with a developing coagulation defect, fresh, whole blood is ideal but is no longer available because of the difficulties of screening for infection (such as AIDS) in donated blood while it remains fresh. A substitute of its component parts should be given as:

- Packed red cells
- Fresh frozen plasma
- Platelets (after 5 or 6 units of blood)

The collaboration of the duty haematologist is important. However, there should be no problem in providing the above, although some haematologists believe platelets are not appropriate. Accurate fluid management with central venous pressure measurement, urinary catheterization and careful fluid balance recording is critical. Serious sequelae develop because of too slow a response to the danger signals.

RETAINED PLACENTA

Correct active management of the third stage of labour involves giving an injection of syntometrine (Syntocinon 5 units plus ergometrine 0.5 mg) intramuscularly with crowning of the head at delivery or with the anterior shoulder. It is then important to exert controlled traction on the umbilical cord with the next contraction to deliver the placenta. It may be difficult to time this correctly if the baby has been placed directly on the mother's abdomen. On some occasions the cord may break or the placenta become firmly trapped above a constricted lower segment. Rarely, a retained placenta is due to abnormal adherence of the placenta to the uterine wall. It is uncommon for excessive bleeding to be associated with retention of the whole placenta, although delayed haemorrhage may be due to retention of smaller parts. It is therefore reasonable, in the absence of pre-existing epidural anaesthesia, to wait an hour or so whilst blood is prepared and operating theatre arrangements made. Vigorous efforts to extract a placenta are painful for the patient, possibly resulting in shock. However, prior to administration of the general anaesthetic after the interval, a brief check should be made to see if the placenta has descended into the vagina.

Insertion of the hand into the uterus requires a strong wrist and forearm! Care should be taken that the fundus is empty. Liberal use of antiseptic cream is desirable. After the placenta has been extracted, an injection of ergometrine is given. Prophylactic antibotics should be given after the procedure.

20

Pregnancy-induced Hypertension (Pre-eclampsia and Eclampsia)

Hypertensive disease of pregnancy is a serious cause of maternal and fetal loss. This includes several conditions in which elevated maternal blood pressure is the most consistent sign. Whatever the cause, significantly elevated blood pressure is taken seriously. However, this section is limited to the management of classical pre-eclampsia and eclampsia. That is a significantly, progressively elevated blood pressure with moderate to heavy proteinuria and fluid retention usually occurring between 24 and 34 weeks of gestation. The following are recognised associates of this condition:

- Nulliparity
- Youth
- Multiple pregnancy
- Polyhydramnios
- Diabetes mellitus

There is a clinical association with poor fetal growth and placental abruption when the disease is severe. Whilst blood pressure can be controlled with medication, the cause of this disease is unknown and the only cure is delivery. The patient with the following symptoms usually has severe disease:

- Severe headache
- Visual disturbance
- Epigastric or right upper quadrant pain
- Tremulousness
- Altered sensorium

Marked symptoms characterize imminent eclampsia. The severe pre-eclamptic usually has heavy proteinuria (greater than 1 g, sometimes more than 5 g), becomes progressively hyperreflexic, and may have a grand mal convulsion (eclampsia); the untreated blood pressure is usually at least 160/110 mmHg.

The following are the cornerstones of management of severe pre-eclampsia and eclampsia.

- Antihypertensive drugs i.v.

- Anticonvulsant drugs i.v.
- Scrupulous fluid balance with urinary catheterization
- Delivery
  Diuretics generally have no place in treatment.

ANTIHYPERTENSIVE THERAPY

Hydralazine is a well tried agent under these circumstances. It is a direct acting vasodilator, exerting its effect principally on the arterioles. It produces a fall in peripheral resistance and a decrease in arterial blood pressure, effects which induce a sympathetic tachycardia. 5 mg is given as a loading bolus by slow intravenous injection over 5 minutes. If a diastolic pressure of 95 mmHg is not achieved within 20 minutes of the injection, a further 5–10 mg is given until this is so. For maintenance, a further injection may be given whenever the diastolic pressure rises above 105 mmHg or a continuous infusion given. 80 mg is then added to 1 litre of sodium chloride (0.9%) for maintenance continuous infusion. Dextrose should not be used as the vehicle. The maintenance infusion is then titrated against maternal blood pressure to achieve a diastolic pressure of 95 mmHg. The principle that the rate of this infusion requires regulation independent of the anticonvulsant therapy is important. Hydralazine should not be used intramuscularly.

In very resistant cases of severe hypertension in pregnancy it may be necessary to resort to the use of diazoxide.

ANTICONVULSANT THERAPY

Chlormethiazole 0.8% (Heminevrin) and *diazepam* (Diazemuls) are effective anticonvulsants. Both are infused initially at a rapid rate to sedate the patient. The infusion is then maintained at a rate which renders the patient drowsy but not unconscious. Unfortunately, both preparations cross the placenta causing significant hypotonia, hypothermia and drowsiness in the newborn. If the rate of infusion is not carefully controlled, the patient may become unconscious with risks of aspiration of stomach contents if the cough reflex has been suppressed. Intensive nursing care is important. Some specialists are unhappy with this state of affairs and have sought alternative regimens such as magnesium sulphate (see below).

FLUID BALANCE

Fluid therapy must be carefully controlled in these patients, who are at risk of renal failure. Urinary catheterization and hourly measurement with a burette is important. The retained fluid in these cases goes to the extravascular space. The circulating volume is depleted and diuretics are contraindicated. If oliguria becomes a problem, then central venous pressure measurement and infusion should be undertaken and an attempt made to expand the intravascular space.

DELIVERY

In severe pre-eclampsia and eclampsia, unless labour is spontaneous and rapid, caesarean section is the better option. It is uncommon to find a favourable cervix at 30 weeks in a nulliparous patient.

MAGNESIUM SULPHATE

In several notable areas of obstetrics there have been obvious transatlantic differences difficult to explain other than by tradition or prejudice. Magnesium sulphate has been used throughout the United States as an effective anticonvulsant in pre-eclampsia. In particular, Gant at Parkland Memorial Hospital, Dallas, has used it as the preferred agent for 20 years in large numbers of patients. Meanwhile, it has been used little if at all in the United Kingdom.

Over the last 2 years, at Kings College Hospital, we have gained experience in its use and have been impressed. One problem is that staff unfamiliar with a method are reluctant to use it in a high-risk situation; thus a self perpetuating cycle remains unbroken. A major concern has been that the therapeutic range is narrow and great care must be taken to achieve the correct dose.

Magnesium sulphate is the preferred agent because:
1 It controls and prevents seizures
2 The patient is alert and awake
3 Airway problems and aspiration are unlikely
4 The fetus is not further jeopardized by heavy sedation.

Any therapy, including this one, is used when a diastolic blood pressure of greater than 100 mmHg is sustained, proteinuria is + + or greater, hyperreflexia is evident. Such circumstances are often also indicative of the need for delivery, which is arranged concurrently.

Intramuscular route

- 10 g magnesium sulphate into each buttock.
- 5 g intramuscularly into alternate buttocks at four-hourly intervals providing the reflexes are still present, the respiratory rate is greater than 16 breaths per minute and the urine output exceeds 100 ml since last dose. The disadvantage of intramuscular therapy is that it is painful and there is a risk of damage to the sciatic nerve. The advantage is that it is more easily controlled and overdosage is less likely.

Intravenous route

- 4 g of magnesium sulphate (20 ml of 20% solution) over 5 minutes.
- Infusion of 20 g in 1 litre of normal saline at a rate of 1 g per hour. Continue the infusion at this rate unless the knee jerks are abolished, urine output less than 50 ml per 2 hours, respiratory rate less than 16 breaths per minute.

Magnesium levels

The normal concentration of magnesium in the serum is 1.5 to 2 milliequivalents per litre (mEq/l). During magnesium sulphate therapy the level rises to 3.5–5 mEq/l. When the concentration of magnesium in plasma rises above 7 mEq/l, signs of maternal toxicity appear. The knee jerk reflex disappears at magnesium concentrations of 7–10 mEq/l. Respiratory depression and, later, respiratory arrest occur at 10 to 15 mEq/l. Cardiac arrest ensues if the magnesium concentration reaches approximately 30 mEq/l. These degrees of maternal toxicity are virtually impossible to reach when the drug is administered carefully and renal function is adequate. Meticulous control of the infusion is necessary. The antidote to magnesium is 1 g of calcium gluconate (10 ml of 10% solution) over 3 minutes. Although decreased urine output referred to previously is an indication for reducing the rate of magnesium infusion, it should be remembered that most postpartum patients, especially those delivered by cesarean section, will have a tendency to be short of fluid and therefore have depleted intravascular volume. Central venous pressure monitoring is a valuable adjunct in this situation.

Magnesium has only a minimal antihypertensive action and an antihypertensive such as hydralazine or labetalol should be given at the same time.

ECLAMPSIA

The management of eclampsia is similar to pre-eclampsia but the fit should be controlled by immediate intravenous therapy. The airway must be secured and oxygen given as first-aid measures. One should not be misled by a normal blood pressure just after a fit. Urine testing will show proteinuria and the blood pressure will rise again in the subsequent few hours. It is important to stabilize the condition before delivery is undertaken, and allow the mother to recover from the metabolic result. This will take 4 to 8 hours.

Although hypertensive disease of pregnancy is associated with serious maternal mortality and morbidity, management as outlined should lead to a successful outcome. Extraneous stimuli should be kept to a minimum, but the intensive care necessary cannot be undertaken in a darkened room. Failure to recognize cyanosis may have serious consequences.

21

Cord Problems

Cord presentation is diagnosed when the umbilical cord is found at the internal os and the membranes remain intact. When the membranes rupture there is cord prolapse. These conditons are associated with malpresentation, abnormal lie, prematurity, polyhydramnios and artificial rupture of the membranes. Although cord accidents are serious most fetuses which are well grown can be saved when the diagnosis has been made soon after the event. When the umbilical cord is being compressed, even in the absence of presentation or prolapse, a typical pattern of variable decelerations occurs on the fetal heart tracing. This is typically seen when there is oligohydramnios and no cushioning effect of the amniotic fluid.

Treatment depends on whether the fetus has succumbed. This can be established by feeling for pulsation in the cord and, in doubtful cases, by performing an ultrasound scan of the fetal heart. If the fetus is dead and the lie longitudinal, then vaginal delivery should be anticipated. Oxytocin is given according to standard indications. A dead fetus in a transverse lie would be delivered in this country by caesarean section, however, skilful internal manipulation and extraction might be performed in a developing country to avoid scarring the uterus.

If the fetus is alive and vaginal delivery not imminent then:
1 Replace the cord in the vagina.
2 Position patient in knee–chest or exaggerated Simm's position.
3 Push head off cord digitally.
4 Perform immediate caesarean section.
   If vaginal delivery is imminent then:
1 Encourage vigorous expulsive efforts.
2 Perform forceps delivery.

The outcome depends on how long the cord has been prolapsed before the diagnosis is made. Exposure of the cord to the atmosphere causes constriction of the umbilical vessels and subsequent asphyxia. Patients admitted with the cord already outside the vulva are more likely to suffer fetal loss. A normally grown fetus is better able to withstand the acute insult than one suffering from intrauterine growth retardation. Cord prolapse occurring in a mature pregnancy in hospital usually has a good outcome.

22

Hepatitis and Acquired Immune Deficiency Syndrome (AIDS)

Hepatitis and AIDS might be seen as *the* infectious diseases of the late twentieth century. Both pose a serious threat to mother, baby and medical staff. Hepatitis causes cirrhosis, liver failure and hepatocellular carcinoma to a considerable degree worldwide, whilst the tragic effects of AIDS are recognized in an increasing number of countries. What is written about AIDS rapidly becomes out of date. So far serious effects of AIDS have been limited to high-risk groups and it may be a decade before it is clear to what extent the general population will be affected. Both conditions require identification of risk groups, blood testing, assessment of infectivity, special precautions, treatment as an inpatient and specific treatment for the baby.

HEPATITIS

Acute hepatitis in pregnancy is uncommon and is managed in conjunction with medical specialists. Asymptomatic carriage of hepatitis antigens is the main concern in pregnant women. The aim is to interrupt and prevent vertical transmission to the child and to protect medical staff. The following are high-risk groups and should be tested:
- Patients from South East Asia, Central Africa, Arabia and the Indian subcontinent. (A group at special risk in the United Kingdom are Vietnamese immigrants.)
- Renal and liver unit patients (status usually known).
- Intravenous drug abusers.
- Residents in long stay institutions.
- Patients with previous unexplained jaundice.

Infectivity is assessed by blood testing. Until the result is known the blood is taken in the pathology laboratory assuming risk. Being hepatitis surface antigen (Australia antigen) positive in itself does not indicate high infectivity. Those who are surface antigen positive should be tested for 'e' status. Those who possess 'e' antigen but no 'e' antibody are highly infectious. The possession of 'e' antibody confers protection. Those of low infectivity should be managed as other delivering patients; gown and gloves with *no* barrier nursing.

High infectivity

Women who are 'e' antigen positive present a problem. Further blood specimens are preferably taken by trained technicians wearing gloves, preventing spillage and appropriately wrapping containers. Childbirth and vaginal examination are particularly high-risk times because of exposure to potentially infective body fluids. Vaccination against hepatitis B is available and a pool of midwifery and medical staff should be protected in this way. Such personnel are considered at risk and health authorities fund vaccination. If shift systems allow, protected staff should be available to look after high-risk patients. Whether protected or not, all staff should take the following measures during delivery or exposure to body fluids (including caesarean section and removal of retained placental tissue).

- gown and hat
- double gloves
- double mask
- goggles

If fetal scalp electrodes are used, extreme care should be taken to avoid pricking the finger, and the electrodes should be disposed of afterwards. The use of intrauterine pressure catheters should be confined to those of a disposable nature in view of difficulties in eliminating viral agents from a Gaeltec catheter.

All soiled material should be removed according to established guidelines, the equipment and room thoroughly disinfected and the woman nursed in a single room with barrier precautions. It is important that such steps are not taken when unnecessary, as the woman feels isolated and alienated.

Baby

Although it is impossible to rid the mother of antigen carriage the cycle of infectivity may be broken by treating the neonate. This is done by passive and active means. A paediatric dose of immunoglobulin is given to the baby soon after birth. This is accompanied by vaccination which is repeated at 1 month and 6 months of age. The baby should be followed up carefully by the paediatrician and immunity assessed. The siblings and other family members should be checked and protected as necessary.

Transmission of the virus appears to occur more commonly in some racial groups than others. Information is awaited from areas of the Far East with high incidence; mainland China, South East Asia, Hong Kong and Taiwan. Vertical transmission appears to be commoner in these areas.

Since writing, it now appears that the Department of Health and Social Security will be issuing recommendations on hepatitis B vaccination to include all babies regardless of 'e' status. The World Health Organisation may be recommending a different vaccination schedule of birth, 1, 2 and 12 months which is slightly different to the existing one in the United Kingdom of birth, 1 and 6 months.

AIDS

AIDS is caused by the human immunodeficiency virus (HIV). After the initial spread of the disease, the principal reservoir has been in the homosexual male population especially in the United States of America. Females have subsequently become infected by heterosexual contacts. A particularly worrying phenomenon has been the reservoir in female prostitutes who are also drug addicts. Haemophiliacs have also become affected because of infection transmitted by blood products.

Three aspects of AIDS are of particular relevance in obstetrics:
1 There is no treatment or cure
2 Infected babies may die in the first year of life
3 Spread to care-givers via body fluids is a possibility

As yet we have no idea about the prevalence of the AIDS virus in the reproductive female age group. Screening studies would provide this information. For the moment, the following high-risk groups should be screened for HIV antibody:
- prostitutes
- those known to have relationships with bisexual men
- intravenous drug abusers
- patients from central Africa and Haiti

If seen early enough in pregnancy, termination should be considered as an option because of the poor prognosis for the baby. With a continuing pregnancy, HIV-positive patients should be treated in the same way as highly infectious hepatitis carriers. No vaccination is available for staff, so scrupulous measures should be undertaken during exposure to body fluids. Unfortunately there is no specific treatment available for the baby, who should be kept under surveillance by the paediatrician.

Guidelines have been issued for the screening of breast milk donors for HIV status in view of potential transmission by that route.

Some hospitals have commenced mass screening for HIV in the pregnant population. Currently consent is required from the patient and counselling must be available. Prospective counselling of every patient is very difficult with current resources. Only when the pattern of antibody positivity and disease in the population is known, can more rational measures be instituted.

23

The Obstetric Flying Squad

The obstetric flying squad or emergency obstetric unit (EOU) is available to a differing degree throughout the country. This facility has often been inappropriately used and it must be remembered that personnel travelling in such a squad are drawn from the duty team at the hospital, consequently weakening it.

Only a minority of ambulance officers are trained in intubation and setting up intravenous infusions (I and I trained). The others are not even trained in taking blood pressure. Their instructions are to radio ambulance control when they believe a bleeding patient is too ill to be transported to hospital. They are naturally cautious; blood loss always looks more dramatic than it proves.

The only purpose of an obstetric flying squad is to resuscitate the patient sufficiently to permit transfer to hospital for definitive treatment. Squads therefore carry emergency drugs, oxygen, blood transfusion equipment, group O rhesus-negative blood, and other supplies for immediate resuscitation. It may be very difficult to place an intravenous cannula in a shocked patient. Time then is of the essence, and the presence of an anaesthetist skilled in cannulation technique may be justified.

Time spent summoning and receiving a flying squad on site with subsequent transfer to hospital is often much greater than initial transfer to hospital would have been. On account of many unnecessary calls a system of direct telephone contact between the most experienced person on site and the senior resident at the hospital is desirable. He or she then has full responsibility of deciding whether or not to send the squad. Basic questions about blood loss, pulse rate, peripheral skin temperature and consciousness are certainly important. In general, patients are much better sent in directly. Such liaison with the hospital team is also important in an area where there are significant numbers of home confinements; currently less than 1% throughout the country.

Part 3
Adverse Sequelae
and Audit

24

Perinatal Death

The juxtaposition of birth and death, or death before birth is something that parents and staff find difficult. The management of perinatal death demands great tact and sensitivity. Obstetrics is a discipline which is largely concerned with happy events. However, about one in a hundred couples go home without a baby. There is no formal training in how to handle this but ultimately it is a matter of sensitive communication.

With advances in prenatal diagnosis, second trimester termination of pregnancy is increasingly performed for fetal malformation or abnormal karyotype. Such cases deserve the same consideration as perinatal deaths. Loss of a wanted pregnancy by early miscarriage is also a traumatic event but will not be considered further here. The technical aspects of managing second trimester termination of pregnancy and induction of labour in cases of intrauterine death (IUD) are considered elsewhere (Chapter 10).

ABNORMAL FETUS AND INTRAUTERINE DEATH

In cases of fetal malformation or intrauterine death, the woman, with her partner if possible, should be informed by a senior member of staff as soon as possible. They should be given time alone and in private to digest the information before any further arrangements are made. They are given the opportunity to ask questions and if they wish they can be shown the ultrasound scan with salient features demonstrated. They may want to go home for a short time to make necessary arrangements but usually prefer to stay in hospital when the inevitability of the situation is understood. A single room, sympathetic care and the offer of mild sedation will be appreciated.

The staff who are going to undertake the procedure should meet the woman and her partner, who are informed what to expect, especially in terms of the time involved. All such cases should be managed in a single room in the labour ward or a specially designated unit. A bed in an open gynaecological ward is inappropriate. Labour ward staff come to see this as part of their job, and some who are particularly suited become dedicated to such cases. A minimum number of staff should be involved and unnecessary intrusion kept to a minimum. The woman's immediate family should be able to stay with her constantly. The full armamentarium of pain relief is made available including epidural analgesia if desired. Some women wish to remain awake and in control but more commonly moderate to large dosages of pain relieving drugs are used.

In advance of the delivery itself a plan should be formulated with the parents about what they want to do. They are offered the chance to see, touch and hold the baby but undue pressure should not be exerted upon them. The abnormal baby is wrapped in drapes for this purpose and difficult situations anticipated. The anencephalic or baby with renal agenesis may gasp although having no chance of survival. These babies should initially be examined by the paediatrician to confirm the diagnosis. Subsequently the baby should be returned to the parents or taken to the neonatal unit to die with dignity. Emotionally traumatic situations may arise for both staff and parents when such practice is not adopted. The parents are then left alone with the child as long as they wish. A polaroid photograph is taken of the child which is offered to the parents. If it is not accepted, then it is carefully stored in the case notes folder for possible future use. The staff with whom the parents have developed most trust should discuss the desirability of post-mortem examination. The body is taken to the mortuary and the parents reassured that they can see it at any time they wish even after post-mortem examination. A well performed examination and dressing of the body restores the appearance.

Most hospitals have an administrative officer who advises on arrangements for collection of the body, the funeral and other matters. Medical staff should ensure that the stillbirth certificate and the request for post-mortem examination are completed as appropriate. In some cases, medical staff will wish to attend such an examination.

FRESH STILLBIRTH

The birth of a stillborn baby which has recently died may be the sequel to adverse factors during labour (intrapartum death) or result from a catastrophic event before the onset of labour such as placental abruption (antepartum death). Some information about how long the fetal heart has been absent is important and will have implications for attempts at resuscitation. If the fetal heart beat has been known to be absent for more than 10 minutes before birth, then resuscitation is pointless, but if there has been a profound bradycardia just before delivery then it may be of some value. In cases of painful tense placental abruption, real time ultrasound in the labour ward is useful. There have been intact survivors born with an Apgar score of 0 at 1 minute, and umbilical cord blood gases estimation is indispensable. If resuscitation is insituted, it should not be discontinued until there has been no response for 20 minutes and this should be at the discretion of a senior member of the neonatal staff.

Intrapartum death should be very uncommon in a well organised labour ward. Its incidence should be used as a measure of the effectiveness of intrapartum surveillance. However, as this is reduced, measures should be taken to ensure that neonatal asphyxia with possible sequelae does not increase *pari passu*. The death or compromise of mature, normally formed babies should be assiduously reduced and eliminated.

It is in the maternal interest that a dead baby be delivered vaginally. However, caesarean section may have been undertaken in an attempt to save the baby. In either circumstance, there is little opportunity for the parents to prepare themselves for the dramatic events anticipated. Senior members of staff should be involved, but especially those with time and sympathy to offer. The delivery and subsequent events should be managed as described in the previous section and staff who have been involved in the care predelivery should not withdraw abruptly after the baby is born. They should quietly and gently say a few words to the grieving parents at an opportune moment.

NEONATAL DEATH

Parents may know that the risk to the life of the baby yet to be born is great, or may be completely unprepared. Women who are cared for in the high-risk antenatal ward should visit the neonatal intensive care unit, meeting staff and seeing the equipment. Obstetric and midwifery staff who have been intimately involved prior to delivery should maintain that interest after delivery, seeing the mother and visiting the neonatal care unit regularly. A close liaison in a true perinatal sense is beneficial and neonatal staff review carefully the use of intensive care and life support systems. If such care is withdrawn then a specially designated area of the neonatal unit may be used for supportive and palliative care; soft furnishings and privacy are appropriate. Some patients appreciate the support offered by the presence of a hospital chaplain or other religious figure at this time and baptism may be undertaken in a simple ceremony.

SUBSEQUENT CARE

After the loss of a baby the mother is nursed in a single room and seen regularly by staff. Bromocryptine (2.5 mg tds) is particularly useful under these circumstances to suppress lactation. Early discharge is anticipated with necessary community care organized, the woman is given a copy of the leaflet *The Loss of Your Baby* and the general practitioner and district midwife are informed. A check list such as shown in Table 24.1 may be used.

Table 24.1 Checklist for perinatal death.

	Initials/date
Consultant obstetrician informed	
Consultant obstetrician seen parents	
Consent for post-mortem	Given/refused
Post-mortem request form completed	
Preliminary post-mortem results explained to parents	
Certification arrangements completed	
Parents offered booklet, *The Loss of Your Baby*	
Lactation suppression considered (bromocryptine)	
Postnatal visit date arranged	
General practitioner notified	
Community midwives notified	
Photograph given to parents or in case notes	
Social worker involved	

Staff who have difficulty communicating under such circumstances must not ignore the couple as this may be seen by the woman as a rejection and taken badly. A few words simply to express sorrow is quite enough.

Follow-up after perinatal death should not be rigid, and the conventional 6 week follow up visit may not be appropriate. The woman should be seen by someone she knows, preferably the obstetric consultant and, in the case of neonatal death, the neonatologist. Comprehensive care should be available with the involvement of a psychologist, psychiatrist, social worker and other specialists as appropriate.

As well as producing the booklet, *The Loss of Your Baby*, the Stillbirth and Neonatal Death Society (SANDS) provides an important support service for these patients.

Mortality, Statistics and Data Collection

Mortality can be measured relatively easily, morbidity cannot. Mortality has been falling steadily over recent years and consequently measurement of morbidity becomes more relevant. Audit based on reliable data collection is essential in maternity services. Nationally, data is collected by birth and death certification. This information is published by the Office of Population Census and Surveys (OPCS) as volumes of annual statistics and regular bulletins in the 'Monitor' series. The Steering Group on Health Services Information (chaired by Mrs E. Korner) reported in 1984 on collection of information for management purposes. A report was published which brought together all the items concerning maternity and specified the items of data that should be collected. Regional Health Authorities agreed to collect all the minimum data sets relating to maternity starting in April 1988. How these should be collected was not stated, but a computerized system is desirable.

MATERNAL MORTALITY (WHO/FIGO)

A *maternal death* is defined as the death of a woman while pregnant or within 42 days of termination of pregnancy, irrespective of the duration and the site of the pregnancy, from any cause related to or aggravated by the pregnancy or its management but not from accidental or incidental causes.

Maternal deaths should be subdivided into two groups:

Direct obstetric deaths. Those resulting from obstetric complications of the pregnant state (pregnancy, labour and puerperium), from interventions, omissions, incorrect treatment, or from a chain of events resulting from any of the above.

Indirect obstetric deaths. Those resulting from previous existing disease or disease that developed during pregnancy and which was not due to direct obstetric causes, but which was aggravated by physiological effects of pregnancy.

Obstetrics is unique in that there is a confidential enquiry into maternal death in England and Wales. Deaths have been reported for 30 years with HMSO publications appearing every 3 years. The enquiry is initiated by the Area Medical Officer after a death is certified, and information is sought from all staff involved in looking after the patient with an attempt made to identify areas of substandard care. The term 'avoidable factors' used previously was often misinterpreted to mean that avoiding these factors would have prevented the death. The documentation of fortuitous deaths and late deaths more than 42 days after delivery has now been de-emphasized. The Scottish system is now being integrated with that in England and Wales.

The maternal mortality rate has fallen dramatically in recent years to 8 per 100 000 maternities in England and Wales; the leading causes of death are hypertensive disease and pulmonary embolism. In less developed countries, maternal mortality remains a major problem; in these areas bleeding and sepsis are pre-eminent.

PERINATAL MORTALITY

The following definitions are taken from the WHO/FIGO recommendations.

Birth

Complete expulsion or extraction of a fetus from its mother, irrespective of whether or not the umbilical cord has been cut or the placenta is attached. Fetuses weighing less than 500 g are not viable and therefore are not considered births for the purposes of perinatal statistics. In the absence of a measured birthweight, a gestational age of 22 completed weeks is considered equivalent to 500 g. When neither birthweight nor gestational age is available, a body length of 25 cm (crown–heel) is considered equivalent to 500 g.

Birth weight

The first weight of the fetus or newborn obtained after birth. This weight should be measured preferably within the first hour of life before significant postnatal weight loss has occurred.

Life at birth

Life is considered to be present at birth (22 weeks, see above) when the infant breathes or shows any other evidence of life, such as beating of the heart, pulsation of the umbilical cord, or definite movement of the voluntary muscles.

Live birth

The process of birth when there is evidence of life after birth.

Still birth

The process of birth of a fetus weighing more than 500 g where there is no evidence of life after birth.

Early neonatal death

Death of a live born infant during the first 7 completed days, (168 hours) of life. The WHO and FIGO recommendations also include the following two statements:

1 All fetuses and infants delivered weighing 500 g or more be reported in the country's statistics, whether they are alive or dead. It is recognized that legal requirements in many countries may set different criteria for registration purposes, but it is hoped that the countries will arrange the registration or reporting procedures in such a way that the events required for inclusion in the statistics can be identified easily.

2 Mortality statistics reported for purposes of international comparison should include only those born weighing 1000 g or more principally on facilities or neonatal intensive care. As those born dead before 28 weeks are often not registered, documentation may be irregular. In the United Kingdom the legal requirement is to register stillbirths only at 28 weeks' gestation and later. If a family want to bury a baby born dead at 26 weeks (considered by some to be a miscarriage or abortion), a signed authorization from the hospital is needed; there is no stillbirth certificate. This is appropriately seen as a saving of expense and formality by some families.

Nonetheless perinatal medicine will only move forward by regarding fetuses born between 22 and 28 weeks as potential survivors. The terms miscarriage, abortion and fetus (the product) should be rejected in favour of perinatal death, premature delivery and baby. The RCOG currently recognizes viability at 24 weeks' gestation and 600 g birth-weight. In the UK the commonest causes of perinatal death are low birthweight and congenital malformation. The perinatal mortality rate has currently fallen below 10 per 1000 births. Several Regional Health Authorities have now set up confidential enquiries into perinatal deaths. Already factors are being identified that will lead to changing patterns of care and improved outcome.

LABOUR WARD REPORTS

As well as mortality analysis, labour wards should be able to monitor morbidity and management. Neonatal morbidity is difficult to measure. Birth trauma related to delivery should be taken very seriously; asphyxia is better measured by umbilical cord gases than Apgar score (see Chapter 16).

Rates of induction and stimulation of labour, emergency and elective caesarean section, and use of types of analgesia are all important. Computerization should lead to reliable on-line availability of such statistics. Management policies may then be adjusted, bearing them in mind. Teaching ward rounds, case discussions, perinatal death reviews and meetings to review statistics are all important in this process.

ANNUAL REVIEWS

Statistics in annual reports should form the basis of management policies in any hospital. Such reports reviewed on a sequential basis permit the evolution of care to be observed and modifications made to provide a better service.

Some Interesting
Fetal Heart Rate Patterns

VARIABLE DECELERATIONS

Different types of variable decelerations manifest varying degrees of asphyxial features, particularly slow recovery, abnormal rate between decelerations, and reduced variability. Fig. A1 shows deep variable decelerations, but with

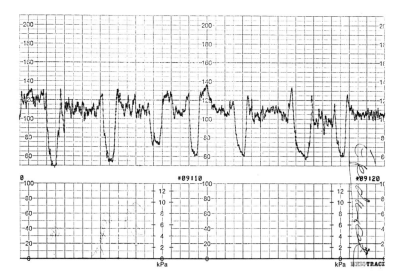

Fig. A1–A11. *Examples of various fetal heart rate patterns.*

quick recovery and good baseline variability between the decelerations, however, the baseline rate is falling gradually. Such a fetus will tolerate this pattern for a short time but will gradually decompensate. Fig. A2 shows deep variable decelerations with good recovery and some pre- and post-deceleration accelerations. Such a fetus has maintained its sympathetic response but may proceed to decompensation. Fig. A3 and Fig. A4 show deep, more prolonged variable decelerations with a reduced variability between them and a baseline tachycardia. This pattern appears as decompensation proceeds to asphyxia. Such a fetus requires delivery soon. Fig. A5 shows the development of biphasic decelerations associated with a hypertonic episode on the contraction trace with an exagerrated post-deceleration acceleration, reduced variability and progressive asphyxia. In summary, well grown normal fetuses tolerate cord compression during normal labour for

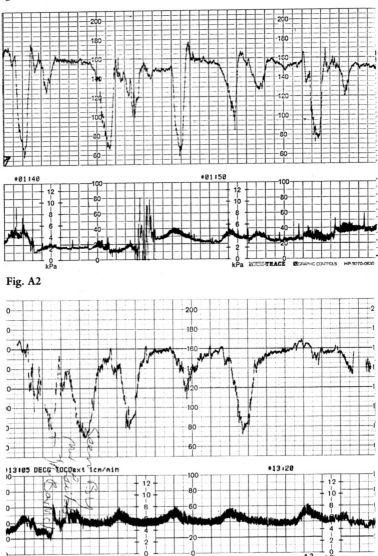

Fig. A2

Fig. A3

a reasonable period of time but when there is a prolonged episode progressive asphyxia develops.

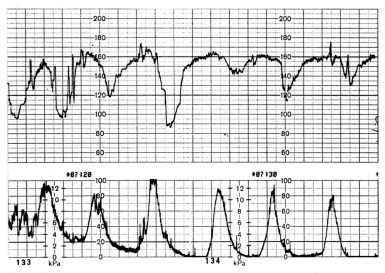

Fig. A4

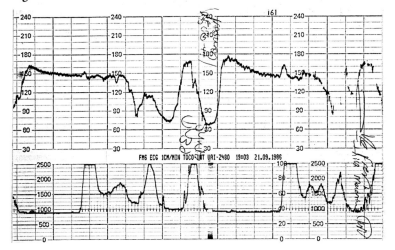

Fig. A5

TWIN FETUSES (Fig. A6)

The latest generation of fetal heart rate monitors, such as the Hewlett–Packard 8040, permits the simultaneous recording of two fetal heart rates on one chart. The heart rate of the leading twin, twin I, recorded from a

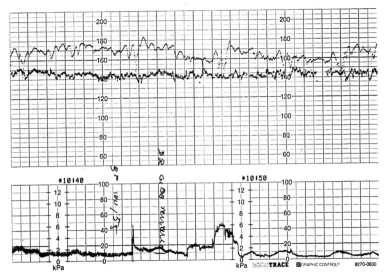

Fig. A6

fetal scalp electrode is the lighter trace. The heart rate of twin II, recorded from an ultrasound transducer is the darker trace. The extreme difficulty of recording three heart rates simultaneously is one reason why labour is avoided in triplet pregnancy: caesarean section being preferable.

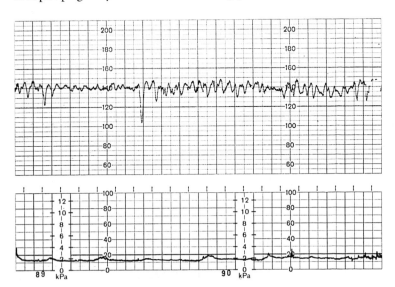

Fig. A7

SINUSOIDAL FETAL HEART RATE

This is a much overdiagnosed condition. If strict criteria are not applied in definition, then many normal fetuses are included who have a pseudo-sinusoidal pattern (Fig. A7). A true sinusoidal pattern shows no short term varia-

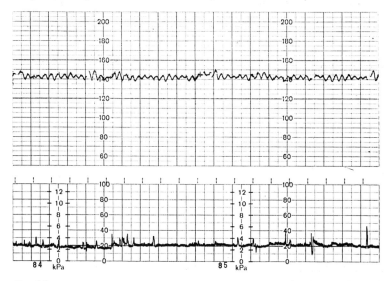

Fig. A8

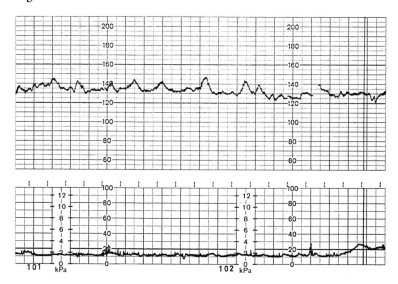

Fig. A9

bility, an oscillatory frequency of 2–5 oscillations per minute and an amplitude of 5–10 beats per minute. There are no accelerations seen. It may be intermittent and is associated with severe fetal anaemia. Fig. A8 shows a sinusoidal pattern in a Rhesus affected fetus with a haemoglobin level of less than 4 g per dl. Fig. A9 shows the same fetal heart rate pattern after an intravascular fetal blood transfusion. I am indebted to Dr Kypros Nicolaides for the above traces.

INTERMITTENT FETAL HEART BLOCK (Fig. A10)

Fetuses that have abrupt changes in fetal heart rate are technically difficult to trace because machines depend upon a series of ECG complexes to generate a trace. The sudden drop in rate can be misinterpreted as a deceleration. Concomitant auscultation or ultrasound scan will provide an explanation.

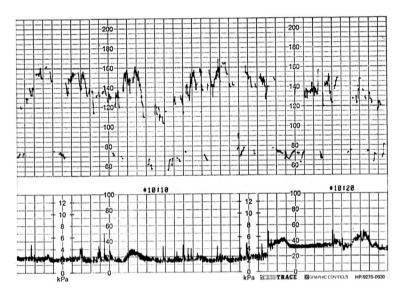

Fig. A10

ARTEFACT (Fig. A11)

This shows a degree of picket fence pattern which should not be mistaken as variability. The electrode should be changed or the wires reversed in the lead.

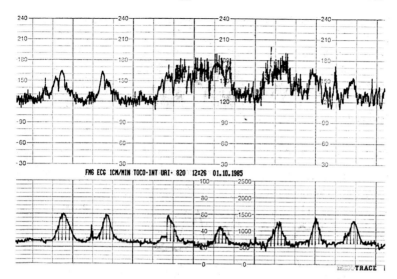

FHG ECG 1CM/MIN TOCO-INT URI- 820 12:26 01.10.1985

Fig. A11

Ultrasonic Fetal Weight Estimation

Fetal weight estimates done using ultrasound depend on reference charts of previously validated fetal measurements compared to weight at birth. Any part of the fetal anatomy that shows constant growth can be used for fetal weight estimate and attention has been focussed on femur length, biparietal diameter, head circumference and abdominal circumference. As a single parameter, abdominal circumference is most relevant. Campbell (1983) constructed the weight prediction by abdominal circumference chart shown in Table A1. Weight estimates can only be expected to be accurate within 10% of the actual weight, and weights at both extremes of the spectrum are least accurate. Large abdominal circumferences do not fit on an ultrasound screen unless a curvinlinear transducer is used. The most widely used calculation, especially for babies of very low birth weight, is the Jeanty and Romero modification of the Shepherd calculation. It uses a combination of biparietal diameter and abdominal circumference as shown in Table A2. Clinicians should always compare their clinical estimate of fetal weight with that determined by ultrasound and, ultimately, with the birth weight.

Table A1 Weight prediction by abdominal circumference.

Abdominal circumference/cm	Weight/kg	Weight/lb-oz (approx.)
20.5	0.84	1-13
21.0	0.90	1-15
21.5	0.95	2-1
22.0	1.03	2-4
22.5	1.10	2-7
23.0	1.18	2-9
23.5	1.25	2-12
24.0	1.34	2-15
24.5	1.43	3-2
25.0	1.51	3-5
25.5	1.60	3-8
26.0	1.68	3-11
26.5	1.78	3-14
27.0	1.87	4-2
27.5	1.98	4-6
28.0	2.08	4-9
28.5	2.18	4-12
29.0	2.28	4-15
29.5	2.38	5-3
30.0	2.48	5-6
30.5	2.60	5-11
31.0	2.70	5-15
31.5	2.80	6-3
32.0	2.90	6-6
32.5	3.00	6-1
33.0	3.10	6-13
33.5	3.20	7-1
34.0	3.30	7-4
34.5	3.40	7-8
35.0	3.48	7-1
35.5	3.57	7-13
36.0	3.65	8-1
36.5	3.73	8-3
37.0	3.81	8-6
37.5	3.87	8-8
38.0	3.93	8-11
38.5	3.98	8-12

Table A2 Estimated fetal weight as calculated from the biparietal diameter (BPD) and the abdominal perimeter.

Abdominal perimeter/mm

BPD/mm	100	105	110	115	120	125	130	135	140	145	150	155	160	165	170	175	180	185	190	195	200	205	210
50	256	266	276	287	298	309	321	334	346	360	374	388	403	418	434	451	468	486	505				
51			285	296	307	319	331	344	357	370	385	399	414	430	447	464	481	500	519				
52			294	305	317	329	341	354	368	381	396	411	426	443	459	477	495	513	533				
53			304	315	327	339	352	365	379	393	408	423	439	455	472	490	508	527	547	568	589		
54					337	350	363	376	390	405	420	435	451	468	486	504	522	542	562	583	605		
55					348	360	374	388	402	417	432	448	464	482	499	518	537	557	577	598	620		
56					359	372	385	399	414	429	445	461	478	495	513	532	552	572	593	614	637	660	684
57							397	412	426	442	458	474	492	509	528	547	567	587	609	631	654	677	702
58							409	424	439	455	471	488	506	524	543	562	583	604	625	648	671	695	720
59									453	469	485	503	520	539	558	578	599	620	642	665	689	713	739

BPD/mm	140	145	150	155	160	165	170	175	180	185	190	195	200	205	210	215	220	225	230	235	240	245	250
60	466	483	500	517	536	554	574	594	615	637	659	683	707	732	758	784	812						
61	480	497	514	532	551	570	590	611	632	654	677	701	725	751	777	804	832						
62			530	548	567	587	607	628	650	672	696	720	745	770	797	825	853	883	913				
63			545	564	583	603	624	645	668	691	714	739	764	790	818	846	875	905	936				
64			561	580	600	621	642	664	686	709	734	759	784	811	839	867	897	927	959				
65					617	638	660	682	705	729	753	779	805	832	860	889	919	950	982	1015	1050		
66					635	657	678	701	725	749	774	800	826	854	882	912	942	974	1006	1040	1075		
67					654	675	698	721	745	769	795	821	848	876	905	935	966	998	1031	1065	1100	1137	1174
68							717	741	765	790	816	843	870	899	928	959	990	1023	1056	1091	1127	1164	1202
69							738	762	786	812	838	865	893	922	952	983	1015	1048	1082	1117	1154	1191	1230

BPD/mm	170	175	180	185	190	195	200	205	210	215	220	225	230	235	240	245	250	255	260	265	270	275	280
70	758	783	808	834	861	888	917	946	977	1008	1041	1074	1109	1144	1181	1219	1258	1299	1340				
71			830	857	884	912	941	971	1002	1034	1067	1101	1136	1172	1209	1248	1287	1328	1371				
72			853	880	908	936	966	996	1028	1060	1094	1128	1164	1200	1238	1277	1317	1359	1402				
73					932	961	991	1022	1054	1087	1121	1156	1192	1229	1268	1307	1348	1390	1433	1478	1524		
74					958	987	1018	1049	1081	1115	1149	1185	1221	1259	1298	1338	1379	1422	1466	1511	1558		
75					983	1013	1044	1076	1109	1143	1178	1214	1251	1290	1329	1370	1411	1455	1499	1545	1592	1641	1691
76							1072	1104	1138	1172	1208	1244	1282	1321	1361	1402	1444	1488	1533	1579	1627	1676	1727
77							1100	1133	1167	1202	1238	1275	1313	1353	1393	1435	1478	1522	1568	1615	1663	1713	1764
78							1129	1163	1197	1233	1269	1307	1346	1385	1426	1469	1512	1557	1603	1651	1700	1750	1802
79									1228	1264	1301	1339	1379	1419	1461	1503	1547	1593	1639	1688	1737	1788	1840

	210	215	220	225	230	235	240	245	250	255	260	265	270	275	280	285	290	295	300	305	310	315	320
80	1260	1296	1334	1373	1412	1453	1495	1539	1583	1629	1677	1725	1775	1827	1880	1934	1990						
81		1367	1407	1447	1488	1531	1575	1620	1667	1715	1764	1814	1866	1920	1975	2032	2090	2150					
82			1402	1441	1482	1524	1568	1612	1658	1705	1753	1803	1854	1907	1961	2017	2074	2133	2193				
83			1437	1477	1519	1561	1605	1650	1697	1744	1793	1843	1895	1948	2003	2059	2117	2176	2237	2300	2365		
84					1556	1599	1643	1689	1736	1784	1834	1885	1937	1991	2046	2103	2161	2221	2282	2346	2411		
85					1594	1638	1683	1729	1776	1825	1875	1927	1979	2034	2090	2147	2206	2266	2328	2392	2458		
86							1723	1770	1818	1867	1918	1970	2023	2078	2134	2192	2252	2313	2375	2440	2506	2574	2644
87							1764	1811	1860	1910	1961	2014	2068	2123	2180	2238	2298	2360	2423	2488	2555	2623	2694
88							1806	1854	1903	1954	2005	2059	2113	2169	2227	2286	2346	2408	2472	2538	2605	2674	2745
89									1947	1998	2051	2104	2160	2216	2274	2334	2395	2457	2522	2588	2656	2725	2797

	255	260	265	270	275	280	285	290	295	300	305	310	315	320	325	330	335	340	345	350	355	360	365
90	2044	2097	2151	2207	2264	2323	2383	2445	2508	2573	2639	2707	2778	2849	2923	2999							
91		2145	2199	2256	2313	2372	2433	2495	2559	2624	2692	2760	2831	2903	2977	3054	3132	3212					
92		2193	2249	2305	2364	2423	2484	2547	2611	2677	2745	2814	2885	2958	3033	3109	3188	3268					
93		2243	2299	2356	2415	2475	2537	2600	2665	2731	2799	2869	2941	3014	3089	3166	3245	3326	3409	3494			
94				2408	2467	2528	2590	2654	2719	2786	2855	2925	2997	3071	3147	3224	3304	3385	3468	3554			
95				2461	2521	2582	2645	2709	2775	2842	2912	2982	3055	3129	3205	3283	3363	3445	3528	3614			
96							2637	2701	2765	2832	2900	2969	3041	3114	3188	3265	3343	3423	3505	3590	3676	3764	3854
97							2694	2757	2823	2890	2958	3028	3100	3173	3248	3325	3404	3485	3567	3652	3738	3827	3918
98								2881	2949	3018	3088	3160	3234	3310	3387	3466	3547	3630	3715	3802	3891	3982	4075
99								2941	3009	3078	3149	3222	3296	3372	3450	3530	3611	3695	3780	3867	3956	4047	4141
100									3002	3071	3141	3285	3360	3436	3514	3594	3676	3760	3845	3933	4022	4114	4207

N.B. All weights expressed in g.
Adapted from the Shephard et al. (1982) equation. From Jeanty and Romero (1983) with kind permission of McGraw Hill.

Further Reading

Apgar, V. (1953) Proposal for new method of evaluation of newborn infants. *Anaesth. Analg.* **32**, 260.

Bishop, E.H. (1964) Pelvic scoring for elective induction. *Obstet. Gynecol.* **24**, 266–268.

Campbell, S. (ed.) (1983) *Ultrasound in Obstetrics and Gynaecology: Recent Advances.* W.B. Saunders, Philadelphia.

DHSS (1979–1981) *Report on Confidential Enquiries into Maternal Deaths in England and Wales, 1979–1981.* HMSO, London.

FIGO (1982) *Report by FIGO Standing Committee on Perinatal Mortality and Morbidity.* FIGO, London.

FIGO (1987) Guidelines for the use of fetal monitoring. FIGO news. *Int. J. Gynaecol. Obstet.* **25**, 150–167.

Flint, C. & Poulengeris, P. (1986) *The 'Know Your Midwife' Report.* South West Thames Regional Health Authority and Wellington Foundation, London.

Friedman, E.A. (1954) The graphic analysis of labour. *Am. J. Obstet. Gynecol.* **Dec.** 1954, 1568–1575.

Gibb, D.M.F. & Arulkumaran, S. (1987) Assessment and management of uterine contractions. *Baillieres Clinical Obstetrics and Gynaecology* **1**(1) 111–129.

Hendricks, C.H. (1983) Second thoughts on induction of labour. *Prog. Obstet. Gynaecol.* 1983, 101–112.

Hendricks, C.H., Brenner, W.E. & Kraus, G. (1970) Normal cervical dilatation pattern in late pregnancy and labour. *Am. J. Obstet. Gynecol.* **7**, 106.

Ingemarsson, I. & Arulkumaran, S. (1985) Beta receptor agonists in current obstetric practice. In: *Recent Advances in Perinatal Medicine* (Chiswick, M.L., ed.), pp. 39–58. Churchill Livingstone, Edinburgh.

Klavan, M., Laver, A.T. & Boscola, M.A. (1977) *Clinical Concepts of Fetal Heart Rate Monitoring.* Hewlett Packard Ltd.

O'Driscoll, K. & Meagher, D. (1986) *Active Management of Labour.* Bailliere Tindall, Eastbourne.

Philpott, R.H. & Castle, W.M. (1972) Cervicographs in the management of labour in primagravidae. *J. Obstet. Gynaecol. Brit. Comm.* **79**, 592–605.

RCOG (1985) *Report on Fetal Viability and Clinical Practice*. Royal College of Obstetricians and Gynaecologists, London.

RCOG (1985) *Report of the RCOG Working Party on the Management of Perinatal Deaths*. Royal College of Obstetricians and Gynaecologists, London.

RCOG (1987) *Report of the RCOG Information and Computing Sub-committee on the Computerization of Maternity Information: How to Cope with Korner*. Royal College of Obstetricians and Gynaecologists, London.

Schifrin, B.S. (1979) The rationale for antepartum fetal heart rate monitoring. *J. Reprod. Med.* **23**(5), 213–221.

Steer, P.J. (1977) The measurement and control of uterine contractions. In: *The Current Status of Fetal Heart Rate Monitoring and Ultrasound in Obstetrics*. Royal College of Obstetricians and Gynaecologists, London, p. 48.

Studd, J.W.W. (ed.) (1985) *The Management of Labour*. Blackwell Scientific the management of primagravid labour. *Br. Med. J*, **4**, 451–455.

Studd, J.W.W. (ed.) (1985) *The Management of Labour*. Blackwell Scientific Publications, Oxford.

Studd, J.W.W., Cardozo, L. & Gibb, D.M.F. (1982) The management of spontaneous labour. In: *Progress Obstetrics and Gynaecology*, vol. 2 (J.W.W. Studd, ed.), pp. 60–72. Churchill Livingstone, Edinburgh.

Index

Page numbers in *italic* refer to figures and/or tables

Index